Vascular Surgery: Questions and Answers

Susanne Regus

Vascular Surgery: Questions and Answers

1000 Facts for the Vascular Surgery Board Examination

Springer

Susanne Regus
University Hospital Regensburg
Regensburg, Germany

ISBN 978-3-662-73386-8 ISBN 978-3-662-73387-5 (eBook)
https://doi.org/10.1007/978-3-662-73387-5

Translation from the German language edition: "Gefäßchirurgie Fragen und Antworten" by Susanne Regus, © Der/die Herausgeber bzw. der/die Autor(en), exklusiv lizenziert an Springer-Verlag GmbH, DE, ein Teil von Springer Nature 2023. Published by Springer Berlin Heidelberg. All Rights Reserved.

This book is a translation of the original German edition "Gefäßchirurgie Fragen und Antworten" by Susanne Regus, published by Springer-Verlag GmbH, DE in 2023. The translation was done with the help of an artificial intelligence machine translation tool. A subsequent human revision was done primarily in terms of content, so that the book will read stylistically differently from a conventional translation. Springer Nature works continuously to further the development of tools for the production of books and on the related technologies to support the authors.

This Springer imprint is published by the registered company Springer-Verlag GmbH, DE, part of Springer Nature.
The registered company address is: Heidelberger Platz 3, 14197 Berlin, Germany

Preface

The idea to write this book arose from daily interactions with final-year medical students and resident physicians training to become vascular surgeons. I repeatedly notice that, although a great deal of factual knowledge is acquired during medical school, applying this knowledge practically to clinical situations and examination settings often proves challenging.

Who hasn't experienced this: you enter your clinical routine full of drive, feel thoroughly prepared, have checklists ready for every conceivable situation, and then suddenly find yourself "drawing a complete blank" as soon as an unexpected question seems to throw everything into confusion. This also becomes apparent in exam situations, when factual knowledge is challenged by critical follow-up questions.

Listing facts and key points is a major strength of us physicians, because we learn it from the very beginning of our studies and later specialist training (we have to). We study with logically organized and tabulated learning materials. However, the subsequent application and understanding of these facts rarely occurs in a logically ordered sequence, but rather in an unstructured, mixed-up manner, arising from the specific situation. This is typical and characteristic of everyday clinical practice. It can be compared to a toddler learning their native language: first, the most important words are learned, then more are added, until eventually simple sentences can be formed. This playful and practically oriented way of learning does not require tables and chapters, but simply continuous learning and application in daily life.

The purpose of this book is therefore to provide a supplement to strictly organized factual knowledge. The concept is to address specific issues that frequently arise in clinical practice, thereby supplementing and interlinking existing knowledge and enabling a better understanding of interrelationships.

The book is intended both for beginners in vascular surgery (laypersons) and for colleagues who are about to take their specialist examination. Here, one can test their knowledge in a playful way and become curious about further insights. Even for me, there were numerous moments while writing when I looked things up and learned something new, which has helped me in my daily clinical practice (and still does).

This book was written alongside my full-time professional work, which is why I got into the habit of writing for 30 min each morning and evening at set times. Often enough, I had to interrupt my writing "in the middle of things" when the time limit was up, only to continue in the evening or the next day. Nevertheless, I was surprised by how much I could accomplish in 2 × 30 min each day. True to the saying: constant dripping wears away the stone. Ideally, this book can serve as a companion long before the looming specialist examination, much like an Advent calendar. Anyone who invests a limited amount of time each day (e.g., 30 min or one question per day) will quickly be surprised by the impact on their individual knowledge base and clinical practice.

I wish all readers and learners much enjoyment and new insights. Both positive feedback and constructive criticism are always welcome.

Ansbach, June 2023 Susanne Regus

Contents

About the Author

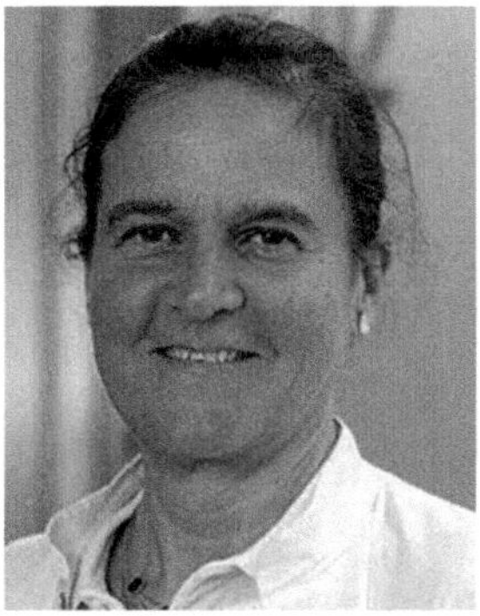

Prof Dr. med. Susanne Regus Vascular surgery, sports medicine, and teaching are passions of the author that extend far beyond her professional life. This is reflected in works already completed and forms the basis for future textbook projects.

Ansbach Clinic, Escherichstraße 1, 91522 Ansbach

Abbreviations

AA	Abdominal angina
AAA	abdominal aortic aneurysm
AAS	acute aortic syndrome
ABI	Ankle brachial index
ACA	Anterior cerebral artery
ACAS	asymptomatic carotid atherosclerosis trial
ACC	Common carotid artery
ACCESS HD	Comparing Catheters to Fistulas in Elderly Patients Starting Hemodialysis
ACE	External carotid artery
ACI	Internal carotid artery
ACM	Middle cerebral artery
ACST-1	asymptomatic carotid surgery trial
AEI	Acute limb ischemia
AFC	Common femoral artery
AFS	Superficial femoral artery
AGE	advanced glycation end products
AHT	Arterial hypertension
AIC	Common iliac artery
AIE	External iliac artery
AII	Internal iliac artery
AMI	Inferior mesenteric artery
AMS	Superior mesenteric artery
Apop	Popliteal artery
AR	Absolute risk
AS	Subclavian artery

ASS	Acetylsalicylic acid
AV	Vertebral artery
AVF	arteriovenous fistula
AVG	Arteriovenous graft
bEVAR	branched endovascular aortic repair
BMT	Best medical treatment
C&S	Crossectomy and stripping
CAS	Carotid artery stenting
CCL	Compression classes
CEA	Carotid endarterectomy
COPD	Chronic obstructive pulmonary disease
Cor	Class of recommendation
CTA	Computed Tomographic Angiography
CVC	Central venous catheter
CVI	Chronic venous insufficiency
DEB	Drug-eluting balloons
DFS	Diabetic foot syndrome
DIGG	German Institute for Vascular Medical Health Research
DPN	Diabetic polyneuropathy
DSA	Digital subtraction angiography
ECST	European Carotid Surgery Trial
EDS	Ehlers-Danlos syndrome
EEA	Eversion endarterectomy
EEG	Electroencephalogram
EKG	Electrocardiogram
ELT	Endoluminal laser therapy
ELV	Endoluminal procedures
ESVS	European Society of Vascular Surgery
EVAR	Endovascular aortic repair
EVLA	Endovenous laser ablation
fEVAR	fenestrated endovascular aortic repair
FMD	Fibromuscular dysplasia
Fr	French
HASE	Hemodialysis Access Surveillance Evaluation
HAV	human acellular vessels
Herz-Echo	Cardiac echocardiography
HHV-8	Human herpesvirus 8
HIV	Human immunodeficiency virus

IE	International unit
IFU	Instructions for use
IMH	Intramural hematoma
INR	International normalized ratio
IONM	intraoperative neuromonitoring
IVUS	intravascular ultrasound
KHK	Coronary heart disease
KI	Artificial Intelligence
KM	Contrast agents
LA	Arcuate ligament
LDS	Loeys-Dietz syndrome
LE	Pulmonary embolism
Loe	Level of evidence
LZ-EKG	Long-term electrocardiogram
MACE	Major adverse cardiovascular events
MALE	Major adverse limb events
MKS	Medical compression stockings
MRA	Magnetic resonance angiography
MRT	Magnetic resonance imaging
NASCET	North American Symptomatic Carotid Endarterectomy Trial
NEJM	New England Journal of Medicine
NIHSS	National Institutes of Health Stroke Scale
NIRS	Near-infrared spectroscopy
NKF- KDOQI	National Kidney Foundation—Kidney Disease Outcomes Quality Initiative
NMH	Low-molecular-weight heparins
NNT	Number needed to treat
NO	Nitric oxide
NOAK	New oral anticoagulants
NSF	Nephrogenic Systemic Fibrosis
NSTEMI	Non-ST-elevation myocardial infarction
OR	open repair
PAT	percutaneous aspiration thrombectomy
PAU	penetrating aortic ulcer
pAVK	peripheral arterial occlusive disease
PCD	Phlegmasia coerulea dolens
PCS	Pelvic congestion syndrome
PopA	Popliteal aneurysms

PTA	Percutaneous transluminal angioplasty
PTFE	Polytetrafluoroethylene
PTS	Post-thrombotic syndrome
PU	Polyurethane
PVA	Polyvinyl alcohol
RA	Regional anesthesia
rAAA	ruptured abdominal aortic aneurysm
RCT	randomized controlled trial
RFA	Radiofrequency ablation
RLS	Restless leg syndrome
rt-PA	recombinant tissue plasminogen activator
SEP	Somatosensory evoked potentials
SOPs	Standards of operating procedures
SPACE	Stent-Protected Angioplasty of the Carotid Artery versus Endarterectomy
SVS	Society of Vascular Surgery
SW	Standard wall
TAA	Thoracic aortic aneurysm
TAAA	Thoracoabdominal aortic aneurysm
TAO	Thromboangiitis obliterans
TASC	TransAtlantic Intersociety Consensus
TASC II	TransAtlantic Inter-Society Consensus II Classification
TBC	Brachiocephalic trunk
TBI	Toe brachial index
TBVT	Deep vein thrombosis of the leg
TC	Celiac trunk
TCD	Transcranial Doppler sonography
TEVAR	Thoracic endovascular aortic repair
TFH	Platelet function inhibitors
TIA	transient ischemic attack
TOS	Thoracic outlet syndrome
TW	dünne Wand
UCA	Arterial leg ulcer
UCM	Mixed ulcer of the lower leg
UCV	Venous leg ulcer
VA	Visceral aneurysm
VAA	Visceral artery aneurysms
VAC	Vacuum occlusive

VCI	Inferior vena cava
VCS	Superior vena cava
VCSS	venous clinical severity score
VEGF	vascular endothelial growth factor
VFC	Common femoral vein
VJI	Internal jugular vein
Vmax	Peak velocity
VN	General anesthesia
Vpop	Popliteal vein
VS	Subclavian vein
VSM	Great saphenous vein
VSP	Small saphenous vein
WFVS	World Federation of Vascular Societies
ZVK	Central venous catheter

Diagnostics in Vascular Surgery

1

Question

1. Which statements about the ankle brachial index (ABI) are correct?

a) The ABI is one of the most important non-invasive diagnostic tools in vascular surgery.
b) Values of < 0.9 are considered indicative of critical circulatory disorders.
c) Values > 1 rule out PAD, even if foot pulses are not palpable.
d) For mediacalcific values, apart from sonography, there are no non-invasive diagnostics to rule out PAD.
e) The pole test is a special diagnostic procedure used exclusively in smokers with suspected iliac artery stenosis.

Answers

a) **Correct.** The ABI provides important information about upstream arterial stenoses or occlusions. It serves as a reliable, easy-to-learn and perform examination, especially for follow-up diagnostics after interventional or surgical procedures.
b) **Incorrect.** Normal ABI values range between 0.9 and 1.2. ABI values < 0.9 are considered pathologically decreased, but a critical circulatory disorder is only defined at values < 0.3. Furthermore, mild PAD is defined as values 0.75–0.9, moderate as 0.5–0.75, severe as 0.3–0.5, and critical as < 0.3.
c) **Incorrect.** In medial sclerosis, which occurs especially in diabetics, values > 1 and absolute pressures > 180 mmHg are not uncommon, which is why further diagnostics are indicated in the appropriate clinical context.

S. Regus, *Vascular Surgery: Questions and Answers*,
https://doi.org/10.1007/978-3-662-73387-5_1

d) **Incorrect.** Other non-invasive diagnostic options include the determination of the toe brachial index (TBI), in which the occlusion pressure in the toe arteries is measured. The toe arteries are typically not affected by medial sclerosis, and the evaluation is equivalent to the ABI.
e) **Incorrect.** In the pole test, the patient lies with the knee joint extended, and the leg is slowly raised while the Doppler signal at the foot is monitored until it disappears. At this point, the height in cm from the bed is measured and multiplied by 0.8. This value is then used as a surrogate for the ABI.

Question

2. Which statements about ABI determination in PAD are correct?

a) Determination of the ABI is the gold standard of non-invasive diagnostics.
b) In mild to moderate stenoses and good collateralization, the resting ABI may be normal and only decrease after exercise (ergometer, treadmill).
c) In diabetics, ABI values can be > 0.9 despite the presence of stenoses.
d) The pole test can only be performed in mobile patients.
e) An ABI value > 1.4 in a patient without diabetes mellitus and without symptoms of PAD 1.4 is of no significance and can be ignored.

Answers

a) **Correct.** As mentioned above, determining the ABI is a simple and quick diagnostic procedure that provides an initial overview of the vascular situation and, if abnormalities are found, justifies further diagnostics.
b) **Correct.** During exercise, there is a physiological increase in muscle perfusion, especially after the end of exercise and if relative ischemia occurred during exertion. Therefore, a drop in ABI to < 0.66 after exercise is an indication of arterial stenoses that are well compensated at rest.
c) **Correct.** Diabetics often have medial sclerosis, especially in the lower leg arteries. As a result, the arteries are not compressible and the occlusion pressures are typically > 220 mmHg, even if upstream stenoses are present. In such cases, it should be documented that the occlusion pressures are altered due to medial sclerosis and are therefore not usable. Caution is advised in diabetics who have an ABI of 0.9–1.2 despite the presence of arterial stenoses. In such cases, determining the toe pressure values (TBI, toe-brachial index) can be helpful.
d) **Incorrect.** The principle of the pole test is that the occlusion pressure at the foot is determined without a tourniquet. This may be indicated, for

example, in cases of medial sclerosis for further diagnostics. The pencil probe is placed on the dorsalis pedis artery, then the leg, with the knee joint extended, is passively flexed at the hip and the foot is raised until the Doppler signal disappears. The distance of the foot from the bed (in cm, e.g., 90 cm) is then multiplied by 0.8. This gives an estimated occlusion pressure in mmHg (in this example, 72 mmHg). This value can then be divided by the systolic pressure at the arm to determine the ABI.

e) **Incorrect.** Several studies have shown that the risk of vascular and cardiovascular events is significantly increased in patients with an ABI > 1.4, regardless of whether the patient has diabetes mellitus or not. Consequently, even in asymptomatic patients, cardiovascular screening should be recommended, and at least laboratory and urine tests should be performed to rule out previously undiagnosed diabetes mellitus.

Question

3. Which of the following is correct regarding Doppler pressure measurement in vascular surgery?

a) In Doppler sonography, ultrasound waves of different frequencies are emitted.
b) The penetration depth in Doppler sonography with a 4-MHz probe is between 3 and 8 cm.
c) The angle of the pencil probe placed on the skin should be < 45° to the longitudinal axis of the artery being examined.
d) When determining the ABI, the lowest measured value at the foot (ADP or ATP) is divided by the highest value at the arm (ABR).
e) The absolute pressure values at the foot play no role in the assessment of circulatory disorders.

Answers

a) **Correct.** Ultrasound waves of different frequencies are emitted. The higher the frequency, the lower the penetration depth. Typically, 4-MHz and 8-MHz probes are used.
b) **Incorrect.** The penetration depth of a 4-MHz probe is 25–40 mm and can be used, for example, for examinations of the popliteal artery or carotid artery. The penetration depth of the 8-MHz probe is 10–25 mm, which is why it is preferably used for superficial arteries (foot, wrist, etc.).

c) **Correct.** This is related to the cosine function. When the sound waves strike perpendicularly, they are usually not detectable, which is often observed as a source of error during the examination. An angle of < 60° is desirable.
d) **Incorrect.** According to the recommendations of the American Heart Association (AHA) and the European Society of Vascular Surgery (ESVS), the highest value of a foot artery is divided by the highest arm arterial pressure. The ipsilateral arm pressure is not used, as this would otherwise lead to falsely elevated indices at the foot in the case of ipsilateral supra-aortic stenosis.
e) **Incorrect.** The absolute values in mmHg also provide information about the extent and degree of compensation of an arterial circulatory disorder. In simplified terms, values > 100 mmHg indicate a very well-compensated situation, 80–100 mmHg a good one, 50–80 mmHg a borderline, and < 50 mmHg a decompensated circulatory disorder.

Question

4. Which statements about pulse oscillography are correct?

a) In pulse oscillography, pulse-synchronous volume changes of the extremity are measured and recorded.
b) The evaluation of pulse oscillography is always based on the absolute values at all 4 extremities.
c) In pulse oscillography, a distinction is made between the mechanical and the electronic measurement method.
d) In acral oscillography, volume fluctuations are detected by piezoelectric sensors.
e) The physiological curve of pulse oscillography is dicrotic.

Answers

a) **Correct.** In oscillography (oscillare = to swing), in general, volume changes are measured and recorded. In pulse oscillography, this is done synchronously with the pulse and depends on arterial perfusion.
b) **Incorrect.** In pulse oscillography, evaluation is always performed by side-to-side or longitudinal comparison. Not only the amplitude of the curve in side-to-side comparison is important, but also the shape of the curve, which is physiologically dicrotic (steep rise, narrow peak, incisura on the descending limb).

c) **Correct.** In mechanical (or pneumatic) measurement, cuffs are placed at different points of the extremity, usually thigh, lower leg, and ankle region, inflated to about 80 mmHg (arterial mean pressure), and volume fluctuations are recorded. In the electronic or acral measurement method, small sensors are attached to the acral parts, which also detect and record volume fluctuations.
d) **Correct.** In acral oscillography, the smallest volume fluctuations are detected by piezoelectric sensors attached to the toes. The principle is simple: pressure on piezoelectric crystals generates an electrical voltage proportional to the applied pressure. These voltage changes are recorded (optically), and the curve shapes reflect the arterial perfusion status.
e) **Correct.** The normal curve is dicrotic (from the Greek di = double and krot = beat). The curve shape is generated proximally (supra-aortic branches) by the Windkessel function of the ascending aorta and in the peripheral vessels by peripheral resistance and the intrinsic elasticity of the vessels. In the presence of a proximal stenosis and/or reduced elasticity, the curve flattens without an incisura on the descending limb, which is referred to as an anarchic curve.

Question

5. Which statements about sonography of the vascular system are correct?

a) A triphasic flow profile in the CFA argues against stenoses in the pelvic arterial system.
b) For sonography of the extremity arteries, a mid-frequency (3–12 MHz) linear transducer is usually used.
c) The low-frequency (1–5 MHz) convex transducer is used for abdominal indications, especially aortic and iliac processes.
d) The B-mode image is rarely needed for vascular surgical questions.
e) Compression sonography for the exclusion of deep vein thrombosis (DVT) is very reliable, especially in the lower leg veins.

Answers

a) **Correct.** In a healthy artery without upstream stenoses, a triphasic signal is typically detected. The first phase (forward) corresponds to the systolic inflow, the second phase (backward) is caused by peripheral resistance, and the third (forward) is due to the Windkessel function of the aorta.

b) **Correct.** With the medium-frequency linear transducer (penetration depth approx. 2–8 cm), most vascular surgical questions regarding neck and extremity vessels can be reliably answered. The high-frequency linear transducer (5–18 MHz) has a penetration depth of only 1–3 cm and is therefore excellent for cutaneous and superficial processes (e.g., varicose veins or arteries of the foot or wrist).

c) **Correct.** Low-frequency (1–5 MHz or 2–9 MHz) convex transducers allow visualization of deeper structures in the abdomen, but also of peripheral vessels in cases of obesity. The advantage of the convex transducer is the greater penetration depth, although this comes at the expense of lower resolution compared to the linear transducer.

d) **Incorrect.** The B-mode image (English: brightness) is also an important examination technique in vascular surgery and angiology, providing an overview of structures and adjacent tissue. The amplitudes and depth of the reflected waves are converted into grayscale values and displayed as an image. Incidentally, B-mode is an advancement of A-mode (from amplitude), which was the original method of ultrasound diagnostics. Here, no two-dimensional image was visible, only the amplitudes and height/depth of their reflected tissue structure.

e) **Incorrect.** Compression sonography is a very reliable diagnostic tool for ruling out DVT, especially from the groin to the knee. It is usually easy to distinguish whether the examined vein is compressible or not. If a vein is not compressible, thrombosis is assumed until proven otherwise. Sensitivity and specificity are both over 90%. However, in the lower leg, sensitivity is significantly reduced and is only about 50%. This also applies to experienced examiners and is explained by the fact that the extremity is often swollen and the naturally small-caliber veins in the lower leg (paired) are more difficult to locate and compress.

Question

6. Which statements regarding imaging with iodine-containing contrast agents are correct?

a) Laboratory screening for renal dysfunction is sufficient.

b) Prevention of contrast-induced renal insufficiency in pre-existing dysfunction can be performed on an outpatient basis.

c) For intravenous fluid substitution, NaCl 0.9% is always used.

d) N-acetylcysteine (Fluimucil) is an important part of the preparation for pre-existing renal insufficiency.
e) From a GFR < 30, angiography with contrast agent is contraindicated.

Answers

a) **Incorrect.** Screening for renal dysfunctions that can lead to acute renal insufficiency includes, in addition to laboratory diagnostics, a targeted medical history. Potentially at-risk patients or conditions include operations in the urogenital area, ostomy patients, diabetes mellitus, arterial hypertension, hyperuricemia, and the use of nephrotoxic medications.
b) **Correct.** Preparation can be achieved through oral fluid intake. The patient should ensure adequate fluid intake the day before the examination, and drink at least 500 ml of water on the morning of the examination and within 2–3 h after the examination.
c) **Correct.** All guidelines recommend NaCl 0.9% for hydration. However, study results indicate that administration of full electrolyte solutions is also possible. The recommended fluid amount is 1 ml/kg body weight/h over 12 h or 4 ml/kg body weight/h over 3 h before and after the examination. This corresponds to a fluid volume of approximately 1000 ml before and after the procedure.
d) **Incorrect.** ACC® 600 was previously administered for prophylaxis of a contrast media reaction. It is no longer part of standard preparation, as studies have shown no benefit.
e) **Incorrect.** Even with a reduced GFR < 30, angiography using iodine-containing contrast agents is possible; however, from a GFR < 45, hydration should be performed.

Question

7. Which statements regarding antiallergic prophylaxis before angiography in known contrast agent allergy are correct?

a) An oral corticosteroid should be administered on the evening before and the morning of the examination.
b) Alternatively, intravenous administration can also be performed.
c) Administration of antihistamines should take place immediately before the examination.
d) Administration of H1 and H2 blockers is absolutely indicated.
e) Contrast agent allergies occur with a frequency of 1–3%.

Answers

a) **Correct.** On the evening before the examination as well as on the morning of the examination, oral administration of Urbason® (methylprednisolone) 32 mg (2 tablets of 16 mg each, total 64 mg) is recommended. The time interval to contrast agent administration should be approximately 12 and 2 h, respectively.
b) **Correct.** Alternatively, Solu-Decortin-H® (prednisolone, 1 ampoule 50 mg) can be administered intravenously 6 h before the examination. When administering corticosteroids, it should be noted that administration 3 h or less before contrast agent application is too short and therefore ineffective.
c) **Correct.** It is recommended to administer antihistamines directly before the examination, ideally when the patient is called from the ward or in the angiography suite by the radiologist. Possible preparations include Tavegil® (clemastine, H1-blocker, ampoule 2 mg/5 ml) as well as Tagamet® (cimetidine, H2-blocker, ampoule 200 mg/2 ml) or Ranitic® (ranitidine, H2-blocker, ampoule 50 mg/5 ml).
d) **Incorrect.** The administration of antihistamines is not strictly necessary; in some cases, only the administration of glucocorticoids is recommended. However, studies have shown that the likelihood of a contrast agent reaction can be reduced to single-digit percentages after prior administration of a corticosteroid and additional application of an H1- and H2-blocker. There is evidence that corticosteroid administration alone is less effective and the risk of a reaction to contrast agents is about 15% in this case.
e) **Incorrect.** Allergic reactions to contrast agents occur with a probability of 0.005–0.5%, more frequently with iodine-containing (0.5–0.1%) than with gadolinium-containing (0.005–0.05%) contrast agents. Most (>95%) contrast agent incidents occur within 20 min, which is why monitoring for 30–60 min is sufficient.

Question

8. What is correct regarding the administration of gadolinium in MRA?

a) Gadolinium can be given regardless of renal function.
b) Gadolinium is metabolized by the liver and excreted via the biliary tract.
c) Nausea and vomiting are common side effects of gadolinium.
d) Nephrogenic systemic fibrosis (NSF) is a common side effect after administration of gadolinium.
e) NSF leads to fibrosis of renal tissue.

Answers

a) **Incorrect.** Even and especially in cases of impaired renal function, the administration of gadolinium and further diagnostics using gadolinium-containing contrast agents should be critically indicated.
b) **Incorrect.** Gadolinium is primarily excreted via the kidneys and, with normal renal function, is no longer detectable in the blood after 5–10 min. However, it can also accumulate in certain tissues, for example in the brain or muscle tissue. This side effect must be considered especially in cases of impaired renal function.
c) **Correct.** Typical, though rare, side effects of gadolinium include nausea and vomiting, shortness of breath, and skin rashes.
d) **Incorrect.** NSF is a very rare complication after administration of gadolinium-containing contrast agents. Fewer than 200 cases are documented in the world literature, the vast majority after administration of linear non-ionic gadolinium compounds (Omniscan®). Macrocyclic preparations (Gadovist®) are much better tolerated and release virtually no gadolinium.
e) **Incorrect.** The primary manifestation is the skin of the extremities, where there is symmetrical involvement with skin discoloration and cutaneous thickening. In addition, joint stiffening can occur within a short period (days to a few weeks).

Question

9. Which statements regarding platelet function are correct?

a) Platelet function inhibitors include acetylsalicylic acid, ADP receptor blockers P2Y12, and glycoprotein IIa/IIIb receptor antagonists.
b) The so-called Multiplate® test is an assessment of platelet aggregation ability using impedance aggregometry.
c) The ADP test of the Multiplate® analysis tests the response to clopidogrel.
d) The platelet count is irrelevant for performing the Multiplate® test.
e) The Multiplate® test is a so-called point-of-care diagnostic.

Answers

a) **Correct.** The most commonly used drug for platelet function inhibition in vascular surgery is acetylsalicylic acid, which inhibits cyclooxygenase 2 (COX2) and thereby irreversibly blocks thromboxane synthesis in platelets.

ADP-P2Y12 receptor blockers include the irreversible inhibitors ticlopidine, clopidogrel, prasugrel, as well as the reversible inhibitors ticagrelor and cangrelor.

Abciximab, eptifibatide, and tirofiban are classified as **glycoprotein IIb/IIIa receptor antagonists.**

b) **Correct.** The Multiplate® test is used both to monitor antiplatelet therapy and to identify patients with congenital or acquired platelet function disorders. The test assesses the aggregation capacity of platelets using so-called impedance aggregometry. The principle is as follows:
   - A blood sample rendered non-coagulable with hirudin is injected into a chamber containing two electrodes.
   - The blood is then mixed with various platelet activators. Activated platelets adhere to the electrodes, thereby altering the resistance (= impedance).
   - A response to platelet function inhibitors is assumed if certain reference ranges of impedance (= aggregation capacity) are not reached.
   - In this way, "non-responders" to platelet function inhibitors can be identified.

c) **Correct.** Testing is performed using the following methods/agents: ADPtest (clopidogrel), TRAPtest (global test), ASPItest (ticlopidine, clopidogrel, prasugrel, ticagrelor, and cangrelor), and ADPtest HS (acetylsalicylic acid and clopidogrel).

d) **Incorrect.** If the platelet count is less than https://doi.org/10.0000/µl, the results of the Multiplate® test are not valid. Therefore, a complete blood count must be performed before Multiplate® analysis.

e) **Correct.** So-called point-of-care diagnostics (POC) includes all diagnostics performed at the patient's bedside. Point of care literally means near-patient laboratory diagnostics. Notable features include that patient samples (whole blood, saliva, swabs) do not need to be processed and results are available without significant delay. It is frequently used in intensive care units, but is increasingly being used in outpatient settings as well.

Peripheral Arterial Occlusive Disease (PAOD)

2

Question

1. Which statements regarding the classification of PAD are correct?

a) Peripheral arterial occlusive disease is classified into 4 stages according to Fontaine.
b) The Fontaine classification is primarily used in Europe.
c) The Rutherford classification exists for both acute and chronic limb ischemia.
d) PAD is most commonly localized in the legs.
e) Upper extremity-type PAD is significantly less common than lower extremity-type and accounts for at most 10% of cases.

Answers

a) **Correct.** The classification is based on the patient's symptoms and the resulting treatment planning. *Stage I* means asymptomatic, i.e., diagnostics have incidentally revealed arterial stenoses or occlusions, but the patient is symptom-free. This is usually due to well-developed collateral circulation. Stage II describes exertional pain with walking distance limitation to > 200 m (IIa) or < 200 m (IIb). The distinction between a and b is based on the assumption that a walking distance of more than 200 m is sufficient and justifies conservative treatment. With a walking distance of < 200 m, most people cannot cope, which justifies invasive treatment. However, the decision must be made individually: for example, a 50-year-old mail carrier with a 500 m walking distance may rightly insist on invasive treatment, as

S. Regus, *Vascular Surgery: Questions and Answers*,
https://doi.org/10.1007/978-3-662-73387-5_2

otherwise his employment is at risk. In contrast, a 90-year-old woman with 100 m may well manage for the rest of her life without invasive measures. Stage III involves rest pain and stage IV trophic lesions. Both are also subsumed under the term critical limb ischemia (chronic). Invasive therapy by percutaneous radiological intervention or surgical vascular reconstruction is unavoidable. Otherwise, limb loss is imminent.

b) **Correct.** In America, the Rutherford classification is mainly used, while in Europe the Fontaine classification is primarily applied. Important differences between the two classifications are the subdivision of **exertional pain** (claudicatio intermittens) into two stages in Fontaine (IIa > 200 m; IIb < 200 m) and three in Rutherford (1: mild, 2: moderate, 3: severe claudication symptoms), as well as the ulcers into one stage in Fontaine (IV) and two stages in Rutherford (V: superficial and VI: deep ulcers).

c) **Correct.** The Rutherford classification exists for both acute and chronic limb ischemia. The chronic classification is divided into stages 0–6, the acute into stages I, IIa, IIb, and III. Details of the Rutherford stages: 0: asymptomatic, 1: mild walking distance limitation, 2: moderate walking distance limitation, 3: severe walking distance limitation, 4: rest pain, 5: superficial ulcers, 6: deep ulcers.

d) **Correct.** In 90% of cases, PAD is diagnosed in the lower extremity. The reasons for this are not sufficiently understood. One possible explanation is that the musculature of the lower extremity in humans is usually subjected to much greater strain than that of the upper extremity, and consequently, stenoses in the shoulder-arm arteries are less likely to become symptomatic. The number of undiagnosed cases is probably higher in the upper extremity than in the lower extremity.

e) **Correct.** Upper extremity-type PAD is significantly less common and most often affects the proximal subclavian artery in the sense of a subclavian steal syndrome. The occlusion process is most often left-sided (approx. 70–80%), although the reason for this side preference is unclear.

Question

2. Which statements about risk factors for PAD in Western civilization are correct?

a) Nicotine abuse is one of the main causes of PAD.
b) Lack of exercise can now be neglected due to the so-called “fitness boom”.
c) Age is another risk factor.

d) Young people under 50 are rarely affected.
e) Regardless of etiology, there are different predilection sites.

Answers

a) **Correct.** Although the number of smokers in Germany has been steadily decreasing for 40 years, almost a quarter of the population still smokes regularly and one fifth daily. According to estimates by the Federal Ministry of Health, a further decrease in the number of smokers is expected in the coming years.
b) **Incorrect.** Lack of exercise is still widespread and is one of the most important risk factors for overweight, metabolic syndrome, and cardiovascular diseases. The WHO recommends 150 min of moderate or 75 min of intense physical activity (running, walking, cycling, swimming, etc.) per week. Only one in five adults in Germany meets this recommendation. This is one of the reasons for an international plan for more physical activity (GLOBAL ACTION PLAN ON PHYSICAL ACTIVITY 2018–2030), for which the WHO is taking the lead.
c) **Correct.** Age is an important, non-modifiable risk factor in the development of atherosclerosis. The incidence is less than 1% in people under 50, but at age 70 it is already 15–20%. Life expectancy is significantly reduced in the presence of PAD. Five-year mortality in 60- to 75-year-old PAD patients is 30%, compared to about 10% in the control group without PAD. The 5-year survival rate of a patient with PAD is lower than that of a woman with breast cancer.
d) **Correct.** Younger people under 50 are rarely affected by PAD. The overall prevalence of PAD in Germany is about 3–10%, rising to more than 20% in those over 70. Exact figures for the prevalence in the < 50 age group are not available, but it is estimated at less than 1%. It is also important to note that diabetes mellitus appears to be a decisive risk factor in the 40- to 49-year-old age group, and smoking in the 50- to 59-year-old group.
e) **Correct.** The vessels of the groin region and thigh are probably the most common localization and predilection sites for PAD, regardless of the underlying risk factors. In addition, predilection sites are found at vascular bifurcations, which is due to the hemodynamics and mechanical stress (shear stress) on the intima and endothelium. In smokers, there is often involvement of the aortoiliac segment, whereas diabetics are affected by stenoses and occlusions of the lower leg arteries.

Question

3. Which statements about the etiology of PAD are correct?

a) Nicotine abuse is, after arterial hypertension, the most important risk factor for PAD.
b) There are 4 main risk factors in the etiology of PAD.
c) With strict nicotine abstinence, the risk for PAD can return to the state before nicotine abuse.
d) The etiology can be divided into biochemical-toxic and hemodynamic-mechanical causes.
e) Arterial hypertension in PAD patients is best treated with 2nd generation β-blockers.

Answers

a) **Correct.** Arterial hypertension is the most important or most common risk factor for PAD. Toxins in tobacco smoke cause a biochemical-toxic endothelial injury, with nitric oxide (NO) being the primary target. NO is a volatile gas with a half-life of 2–10 s and diffuses freely through the vessel wall. It leads, among other things, to vascular wall relaxation and reduced adhesion of blood cells, mainly platelets. The components of tobacco disrupt these sensitive regulatory processes, resulting in endothelial deposits. In addition, smokers have increased blood levels of carbon monoxide, which leads to increased vasoconstriction and accelerates the process of "vascular calcification".
b) **Correct.** At least one of the 4 risk factors is present in > 95% of all patients with PAD. These are
   1. Nicotine abuse,
   2. Diabetes mellitus,
   3. Arterial hypertension, and
   4. Hypercholesterolemia.
c) **Incorrect.** Even after consistent cessation of nicotine abuse, the risk for developing PAD does not return to that of lifelong non-smokers, even after years or decades of abstinence. This is a peculiarity of PAD, because in other diseases (CAD, obstructive lung diseases, malignant tumors), the disease risk can completely normalize after quitting smoking.
d) **Correct.** Broadly, the etiology of endothelial and intimal injury, which is characteristic of atherosclerosis, can be divided into mechanical and

chemical causes. Chemical causes include smoking with its harmful components, diabetes mellitus with elevated blood glucose levels, and hyperlipidemia. Mechanical causes include arterial hypertension and anatomical peculiarities at vascular bifurcations.

e) **Incorrect.** Until a few years ago, β-blockers were contraindicated in the guidelines of the German Society for Angiology. First- and second-generation β-blockers, due to their non-selective action, cause not only the desired β1-blockade but also peripheral β2-blockade. This leads to a predominance of alpha action and peripheral vasoconstriction, which can worsen PAD symptoms. Third-generation β-blockers (nebivolol, carvedilol), on the other hand, are selective for β1-receptors and are therefore used and recommended in PAD patients alongside ACE inhibitors, AT-I antagonists, and calcium antagonists.

Question

4. Which statements about the pathogenesis of arteriosclerosis are correct?

a) So-called "fatty streaks" are the first stage of arteriosclerosis and occur in advanced age.
b) "Fatty streaks" are the precursors of atherosclerotic plaques.
c) In atherosclerotic plaques, a distinction is made between early (simple) and late (complex) plaques.
d) Calcifications arise from the breakdown of fat deposits, but only in late atherosclerotic plaques.
e) Arteriolosclerosis is arteriosclerosis of small vessels.

Answers

a) **Incorrect.** "Fatty streaks" are lipid deposits beneath the endothelium that are already observed in childhood. They are completely reversible; only a small proportion of these "fatty streaks" progress to an atherosclerotic plaque.
b) **Correct.** Atherosclerotic plaques can develop from "fatty streaks," which are characterized by a central atheromatous core. This is highly thrombogenic and is separated from the vessel lumen by a fibrous cap.
c) **Correct.** Simple plaques consist of the central atheromatous core and the fibrous cap. Over time, repeated minor and major tears in the cap lead to local partial thrombosis and reorganization of the plaque. Over time,

several layers form, resulting in thickening of the cap and organization of the atheromatous core into multiple layers. This leads to complex plaques, which can typically be seen and removed intraoperatively.

d) **Incorrect.** Calcifications are already observed in early atherosclerotic plaques and can, in principle, occur in all cells with tissue necrosis and metabolic acidosis. Calcifications are thus a consequence of cell death and tissue reorganization. They do not arise from deposition of blood components (e.g., in the context of hypercalcemia).

e) **Incorrect.** Arteriolosclerosis involves deposits of hyaline substances in the vessel wall, usually in smaller arteries (renal artery or dorsalis pedis) and downstream capillaries. These hyaline substances are formed by the attachment of sugars to proteins, fats, and nucleic acids. The resulting substances are also called advanced glycation end products (AGE). The deposits are of rather firm structure, can completely occlude the lumen, and are observed, among other things, in diabetic nephropathy and stenosis of the renal arteries as well as in diabetic foot syndrome with microangiopathic changes.

Question

5. Which statements about the histopathological processes in the vessel wall and their pathogenesis in PAD are correct?

a) PAD mainly occurs in the endothelium and intima.
b) With nicotine abuse, tar and its breakdown products are deposited in the endothelium.
c) In diabetics, glucose and fructose are deposited and induce an inflammatory process.
d) Vascular bifurcations are most frequently affected by atherosclerotic vessel wall changes.
e) In arterial hypertension, tears in the intima occur, leading to an inflammatory reaction of the vessel wall.

Answers

a) **Correct.** According to current scientific knowledge, endothelial cells play the main role in the development of atherosclerotic plaques. Normally, endothelial cells form an inner lining of the vessels that is impermeable to corpuscular components. In atherosclerosis, various mechanisms lead to an inflammatory reaction of the endothelial cells, making them permeable to macrophages and fats. This leads to deposits in the intima, resulting in so-called plaques. Depending on the components of these plaques, they are either "soft" (lipid-rich) or "hard" (calcium- and mineral-rich). As the disease progresses, these plaques increase in size, leading to stenoses or aneurysms. In addition, an inflammatory process is activated, causing inflammatory cells to migrate into the plaques and leading to a certain encapsulation.

b) **Correct.** With nicotine consumption, numerous toxins, poisonous substances, carcinogens, and tar-containing components are inhaled and transported by the bloodstream. These lead to the typical deposits, which in smokers are mainly localized aortoiliacally.
c) **Correct.** In diabetics, the pathognomonic hyperglycemia, which is causative for plaque formation in diabetics, leads to deposits of these excess blood substances. Here, too, an inflammatory process is induced; calcifications are also typical, and due to the usually coexisting overweight, there are also deposits of lipids.
d) **Correct.** Due to blood flow-induced turbulence at vascular bifurcations, there is shear stress on the vessel wall, which is evidently responsible for intimal lesions. These lesions create predilection sites for deposits of excess blood components. A similar situation is assumed for the femoral artery at the level of the adductor canal. Here, too, constant pressure is thought to cause intimal lesions, making this region (loco typico) more susceptible to discontinuities and deposits.
e) **Correct.** Arterial hypertension is also an important risk factor in the development of PAD. The vessel wall stress due to hypertension is also thought to cause tears or lesions in the vessel wall, which then trigger the already repeatedly cited cascade of plaque formation.

Question

6. Which statements about the localization of occlusive processes are correct?

a) In diabetics, the lower leg vessels are most commonly affected.
b) In smokers, the femoral and lower leg arteries are often unremarkable.
c) One of the most common sites of stenosis is the superficial femoral artery (SFA) at the level of the adductor canal.
d) Long-segment occlusions usually affect the SFA, less commonly the popliteal and crural arteries.
e) Short-segment stenoses are often found at bifurcations, mechanically stressed vessel segments, and diffusely in lower leg arteries.

Answers

a) **Correct.** In diabetics, occlusive processes are often found in the lower leg, whereas the iliac and femoral arteries are usually free of stenosis. The cause of these crural stenoses in diabetics is diabetic medial sclerosis.
b) **Correct.** In smokers, stenoses are usually found aortoiliacally, whereas the femoropopliteal segment typically shows normal findings without abnormalities. Smokers are also often younger, between 50 and 60 years old, and less likely to be overweight.
c) **Correct.** The SFA at the level of the adductor canal is a predilection site for PAD. Other predilection sites are bifurcations (carotid, femoral bifurcation, aortic and iliac bifurcation) as well as mechanically stressed vessel regions such as the popliteal artery (popliteal) and the external iliac artery (EIA).
d) **Correct.** Long-segment occlusions often affect the SFA with collateralization via the profunda femoris artery and reconstitution of the popliteal artery above (supragenual) or below (infragenual) the knee joint. Patients become symptomatic only when collateralization is no longer sufficient to ensure adequate blood supply to the leg. Lower leg vessels can also be occluded over long segments, but this rarely affects smokers and is mainly seen in diabetics and elderly patients.
e) **Correct.** Stenoses occur particularly at bifurcations, probably due to the resulting turbulence. This apparently leads to increased deposition of blood-borne substances. The same likely applies to mechanically stressed vessel areas, such as the EIA during hip movement, the popliteal artery at the knee joint, or the SFA at the adductor canal.

Question

7. Which statements about bypasses and bypass materials are correct?

a) The GSV is the most commonly used bypass material.
b) Among alloplastic materials, PTFE (polytetrafluoroethylene) and Dacron prostheses are notable.
c) Allogeneic or homologous replacement materials include, for example, cryopreserved aortas from deceased donors.
d) Among heterologous materials, umbilical vein grafts are notable.
e) The composite bypass is a very promising alternative when the GSV is of insufficient length.

Answers

a) **Correct.** If sufficiently long and with a diameter of > 3 mm, the GSV is the most suitable material for a bypass graft. It has 5-year patency rates of more than 80%. After one year, more than 90% of vein bypasses remain patent. The small saphenous vein and the basilic vein are less suitable and therefore used less frequently.

b) **Correct.** PTFE and Dacron are typical alloplastic materials and are used for arterial reconstructions. PTFE stands for polytetrafluoroethylene (often referred to by the manufacturer names Goretex® or Teflon® prostheses) and is a primarily impermeable plastic with a smooth surface. PET stands for polyethylene terephthalate and is the base material for polyester prostheses (also known as Dacron). These prostheses are knitted or woven, are stretchable, but are not primarily impermeable. In the past, PET prostheses had to be "clotted," meaning they were placed in the patient's blood and made impermeable by the adhesion of corpuscular components. This led to a certain intraoperative time delay, which is why coated prostheses are now available and have become established in clinical practice.

c) **Correct.** Allogeneic or homologous means that these are biological materials from the same species (human), but not from the same individual (autologous), rather from another individual of the same species. Typically, these are larger arteries from deceased humans, most often the aortoiliac axis.

To better remember the sometimes differently used terms, here is a summary:

- auto**genous** (obsolete: autologous): from the same individual
- allo**genous** (obsolete: homologous): from another individual of the same species
- xeno**genous** (obsolete: heterologous): from another species
- alloplastic: not biological material, but synthetic

d) **Incorrect.** Heterologous is an outdated term and synonymous with xenogeneic. This means that it is biological tissue from another species, most commonly bovine pericardium (bovine pericardial patch). The advantage is the significantly lower susceptibility to infection. These patches are now available in different diameters and thicknesses, which is why they are increasingly used in cardiac as well as vascular surgery. However, there is currently no commercial production of tubular pericardial materials that could be used as bypass grafts.

e) **Incorrect.** The composite bypass is typically used when the GSV is not long enough, but due to poor patency rates, it is not a good alternative. In this procedure, the vein is anastomosed to a synthetic bypass to achieve the required length. However, the patency rates of such composite bypasses are unsatisfactory; after 5 years, only about 30% of these bypasses remain patent. Their use is therefore limited to exceptional cases, e.g., to create the distal anastomosis in the lower leg area and the joint-crossing segment with a vein, and then use synthetic material (usually PTFE) in the thigh.

Question

8. Which statements about PAD in diabetics are correct?

a) In diabetics, stenosing processes usually develop in the lower leg arteries.
b) The main cause of arteriosclerosis in diabetics is glucose deposits in the vessel wall.
c) In diabetic macroangiopathy, Mönckeberg's medial sclerosis is most often observed histopathologically.
d) In diabetic microangiopathy, foot pulses are often palpable.
e) In diabetics, the triopathy of angiopathy, neuropathy, and infection plays a central role in the development of foot ulcers.

Answers

a) **Correct.** In diabetics, stenosing processes are often observed in the crural arteries or as microangiopathy in the acral regions. In more than 70% of diabetics, arteriosclerotic processes are localized in the extremity arteries below the knee joint.
b) **Correct.** Chronically elevated blood glucose levels lead to glycation of proteins and corpuscular blood components, which deposit in the extracellular matrix and the vessel intima.
c) **Correct.** Mönckeberg's medial sclerosis is histopathologically characterized by calcifications of the media layer, which are typically long-segment and non-stenosing. Mönckeberg's sclerosis preferentially occurs in the lower leg arteries, but the renal arteries can also be affected. Due to the calcifications of the media, the arteries can no longer be properly compressed, which is why ABI measurement often yields falsely high values.
d) **Correct.** Typically, in diabetic microangiopathy, glycated proteins are deposited in the vessel intima and there is damage to the endothelium of capillaries. This leads to poorer perfusion of the acral regions, in addition

to reduced sensitivity due to perfusion impairment of sensory nerves. This combination of microangiopathy and neuropathy promotes the occurrence of non-healing ulcerations, which are typically found in diabetic foot syndrome.

e) **Correct.** It is estimated that one third of patients with diabetes mellitus will develop diabetic foot syndrome during their lifetime. The causes, in addition to micro- and macroangiopathy, also include the frequently observed neuropathy and infection of existing ulcers at the foot. Since these three mechanisms reinforce each other, the risk of amputation is very high without adequate therapy.

Question

9. Which statements about the ankle-brachial Doppler index are correct?

a) In determining the ankle-brachial Doppler index, the systolic blood pressure at the arm is divided by the occlusion pressure at the foot.
b) An ABI between 0.9 and 1.2 is considered normal and excludes PAD.
c) An ABI of < 0.7 is considered a critical perfusion disorder.
d) In the pole test, the occlusion pressure at the foot in non-compressible arteries (medial sclerosis) is estimated by elevating the leg above heart level.
e) The highest measured value at the foot should always be used for ABI calculation.

Answers

a) **Incorrect.** In determining the ankle-brachial Doppler index, also known as ABI (ankle brachial index), the occlusion pressure of the foot arteries is divided by the pressure measured at the arm. The ABI is one of the most important non-invasive diagnostic methods in vascular surgery.
b) **Incorrect.** The normal range for ABI values is indeed between 0.9 and 1.2, and in most cases, PAD can be excluded on this basis. However, in diabetics, values are regularly higher (keyword medial sclerosis), so PAD cannot be excluded by ABI measurement alone in these cases. In such cases, the pole test and duplex sonography are recommended.
c) **Incorrect.** The severity of PAD based on ABI can be roughly classified as follows:

I. > 1.5 medial sclerosis (not evaluable)
II. 1.2–0.9: normal range
III. 0.7–0.9: mild PAD

IV. 0.5–0.7: moderate PAD
V. 0.3–0.5: severe PAD
VI. < 0.3: critical PAD
However, these are only guidelines that must always be assessed in conjunction with the clinical findings and symptomatology.

d) **Correct.** In the pole test, the patient's leg is slowly elevated above heart level while the flow at the foot is continuously monitored with the Doppler probe. The height of the foot in cm when the signal disappears is multiplied by 0.8. The resulting value (e.g., 100 cm height × 0.8 = 80) is the estimated occlusion pressure in mmHg. If a signal is present up to a height of 75 cm, there is no contraindication to compression therapy or wearing medical compression stockings (for example, in mixed leg ulcers). The critical perfusion pressure is then 60 mmHg.
e) **Correct.** If a signal and measurable occlusion pressure can only be obtained from one foot artery, this value is decisive for the ABI. If a signal can be obtained from two or all three arteries, the highest value is used as the reference for the ABI.

Question

10. Which statements about sonographic screening in PAD are correct?

a) Every patient with a cardiovascular risk profile should be sonographically screened for PAD.
b) Diabetics require regular ultrasound examinations to detect peripheral stenoses at an early stage.
c) After a femoropopliteal bypass, patency should be regularly monitored sonographically.
d) Sonographic follow-up is pointless in an asymptomatic aortic aneurysm with a diameter of 3 cm.
e) In the BASIL study (bypass versus angioplasty in severe ischemia of the leg), secondary patency rates after surgical and interventional vascular procedures could be improved by sonographic monitoring.

Answers

a) **Incorrect.** Sonographic screening in asymptomatic patients is not indicated, even in the presence of a positive cardiovascular risk profile. The reason is the lack of consequences for asymptomatic patients and the considerable time required. Nevertheless, and this is independent of sonographic screening, every patient with a cardiovascular risk profile should be informed about the increased risk of complications and mortality, and "best medical treatment" including lifestyle changes should be recommended.

b) **Incorrect.** Patients with diabetes mellitus do have an increased risk of developing PAD, especially medial sclerosis of small and very small vessels. However, regular ultrasound screening is still not indicated; more important are good blood glucose control and regulation of risk factors. In addition, pressure relief at the foot is necessary to prevent the development or progression of ulcerations.
c) **Incorrect.** According to current studies, regular sonographic follow-up of femoropopliteal bypasses is not indicated, although it may be justified in risk situations (e.g., poor peripheral runoff) and in anxious patients. Nevertheless, the patency rates of regularly sonographically monitored bypasses are no better than those without regular monitoring.
d) **Incorrect.** Sonographic follow-up of aortic aneurysms makes sense from 3 cm or in the case of rapid size progression (more than 0.5 cm in 6 months). Further sonographic follow-up is useful for popliteal aneurysms from a diameter of 1.5 cm and carotid stenoses from a degree of stenosis of 60–70%. In clinical practice, follow-up is often performed for high-risk bypasses to detect anastomotic stenoses early. Sonographic monitoring is also recommended after complex peripheral interventions to detect relevant restenoses early, which is particularly important after stent implantation. Finally, endovascularly excluded aortic aneurysms are also regularly monitored sonographically, increasingly using contrast-enhanced ultrasound as a substitute for CT angiography.
e) **Incorrect.** Subgroup analyses showed no benefit of regular sonographic monitoring on secondary patency rates after either surgical or interventional therapy. This has also been incorporated into the guidelines of the professional societies. Ultimately, it is certainly possible and advisable to perform regular sonographic monitoring, but due to lack of evidence, there are no concrete recommendations or time intervals.

Question

11. Which statements regarding the indication for invasive therapeutic measures in PAD are correct?

a) In principle, invasive therapy should only be indicated when walking distance is limited to less than 200 m.
b) In PAD stage IIb, invasive therapy should definitely be recommended.

c) Superficial ulcers can be safely treated conservatively in multimorbid patients.
d) Nocturnal rest pain is always an indication for revascularization.
e) In a multimorbid bedridden patient with advanced PAD stage IV, arterial reconstructions should be indicated with extreme caution.

Answers

a) **Incorrect.** In individual cases, the indication for invasive, i.e., surgical or interventional, therapeutic measures can be made earlier. The patient's activity level and age should always be considered. For example, patients with gonarthrosis sometimes receive knee prostheses when their walking distance is limited to 500 m, or endurance athletes undergo Achilles tendon correction if their marathon career depends on it. The same should be considered for vascular interventions. Thus, a 50-year-old mail carrier with a walking distance limited to 1000 m should undergo invasive therapy, as should a competitive cyclist whose career is threatened by iliac endofibrosis, even if he is otherwise unrestricted in daily life.
b) **Incorrect.** In the stage of intermittent claudication, the indication for therapy is always relative. The patient's general condition and lifestyle, especially activity level, should always be considered. The 90-year-old woman who manages well in her apartment with a walking distance of 20 m and copes with her daily life usually does not require angioplasty of a stenosed superficial femoral artery or thromboendarterectomy with patch plasty of the femoral bifurcation. Most patients, including their concerned relatives, understand the preference for conservative therapy, especially when the possible complications of an invasive procedure are explained to them.
c) **Incorrect.** In individual cases, superficial ulcerations, especially if they are healing, can certainly be treated conservatively. Nevertheless, ulcerations caused by arterial stenoses or occlusions are, by definition, PAD stage 4, i.e., a critical perfusion disorder. The risk of limb loss is significantly higher here than in intermittent claudication, and this should be communicated to patients. Patients and their relatives should be informed that any increase in ulcerations should lead to a follow-up and re-examination. If there are no contraindications to invasive therapy, it should be recommended and performed.
d) **Correct.** Nocturnal rest pain caused by PAD should prompt revascularization. However, a thorough and differentiated history should also be taken.

Typical of ischemic rest pain is improvement as soon as the patient stands up or lets the legs hang out of bed. Tingling in the soles of the feet, regardless of foot position, is not a reliable sign of PAD and should prompt further investigation. Rest pain with arterial stenoses demonstrated on imaging should, in principle, also prompt extensive arterial reconstruction. Rest pain is, by definition, a critical perfusion disorder associated with the risk of limb loss.

e) **Correct.** In elderly, multimorbid, and bedridden patients, complex arterial reconstructions should only be indicated in exceptional cases. These patients often also have contractures in the hip and knee joints, which is a clear sign of prolonged immobility. In addition, the surgical procedure carries a significant risk of complications, so the potential benefit of limb salvage in an immobile patient is negligible. In these cases, a detailed discussion should be held with the relatives and the patient, explaining and recommending the possibility of conservative or surgical therapy by means of amputation.

Question

12. Which statements about TASC (Trans Atlantic Inter-Society Consensus) are correct?

a) These are recommendations for the treatment of PAD from a vascular surgical perspective.
b) This is a classification of aortoiliac and femoropopliteal PAD based on morphological criteria.
c) The TASC-II classification is relatively up-to-date and is based on available innovative therapeutic options.
d) The TASC-II classification from A to D is based on the severity and morphology of stenoses and occlusions of the arterial axis.
e) The completion of an updated TASC-III recommendation is expected in 2023.

Answers

a) **Incorrect.** The first consensus paper was published in 2000. Various professional societies (including vascular surgeons, radiologists, cardiologists, angiologists) from Europe and the United States participated, with the aim of improving and standardizing the treatment of patients with PAD. Its significance lies in its interdisciplinarity. The first version (TASC) comprised nearly 300 pages and was divided into 3 chapters: intermittent claudication, acute and chronic critical limb ischemia.

b) **Correct.** With the increasing availability of endovascular techniques for the treatment of arterial stenoses and occlusions, the TASC-II classification was developed to provide some structure and guidance in selecting therapy options. A means that endovascular therapy should be preferred, while D is a clear recommendation for open surgical therapy. For B and C, either may be indicated, depending on the expertise and preferred techniques of the practitioner.

c) **Incorrect.** The TASC-II classification dates from 2007 and does not, or only partially, take into account new and innovative developments that have occurred since then. In particular, advances in endovascular therapy and the increasingly improved materials available for it were only marginally considered.

d) **Correct.** The classification of occlusive processes is from A to D, with A representing less severe findings (short-segment, unilateral, rarely bilateral) that should almost always be treated endovascularly. D represents extensive occlusive processes (long-segment, bilateral, involving bifurcations), for which surgical treatment is generally recommended. B and C are intermediate, so decisions should be made individually, taking into account institutional experience and the patient's condition. The trend for type B lesions is toward endovascular treatment, for type C toward open surgical therapy. Hybrid procedures, i.e., combinations of open and endovascular approaches, are also increasingly used.

e) **Incorrect.** The update planned for 2011 (TASC IIa) was withdrawn because the participating experts and professional societies could not reach agreement. In addition, the nature and extent of industry involvement and significant conflicts of interest were criticized. The TASC-III project planned for 2013 failed for similar reasons, which is why the **ESVS** (European Society of Vascular Surgery, representing Europe), the **SVS** (Society of Vascular Surgery, representing North America), and the **WFVS** (World Federation of Vascular Societies, representing Australia, New Zealand, Asia) withdrew from the TASC project. The representatives of the professional societies made this decision by mutual agreement at a meeting in Budapest.

Question

13. Which statements about anticoagulation in PAD patients are correct?

a) After infrainguinal (i.e., femorodistal) bypass surgery, oral anticoagulation should always be performed.
b) Dual antiplatelet therapy should be indicated for all infragenual bypasses.
c) After percutaneous transluminal angioplasty (PTA) of the lower leg (crural), at least temporary oral anticoagulation has proven effective.
d) For infrainguinal bypasses with poor runoff, oral anticoagulation with phenprocoumon is better than the use of NOACs.
e) In PAD patients, after peripheral revascularization, administration of clopidogrel 75 mg once daily for 4 weeks post-interventionally in addition to low-dose rivaroxaban 2.5 mg twice daily and acetylsalicylic acid 100 mg once daily (according to the VOYAGER-PAD study) leads to serious bleeding complications.

Answers

a) **False.** The results of a multicenter randomized study from the Netherlands (BOA: Bypass oral anticoagulants versus aspirin) from the year 2000 showed that femorodistal bypasses should be treated postoperatively depending on the bypass material used. The results under oral anticoagulation (with phenprocoumon) were compared with acetylsalicylic acid. The patency rate of autologous vein bypasses was, regardless of the distal target vessel, significantly better under oral anticoagulation than with administration of an antiplatelet agent. Conversely, synthetic bypasses showed better patency rates under acetylsalicylic acid. This actually contradicts the expectation and the "feeling" of the clinician that synthetic bypasses require "stronger" blood thinning than vein bypasses. Nevertheless, it has proven effective to treat high-risk bypasses (poor runoff, poor vein material, repeat procedures) with oral anticoagulation. For vein bypasses without the aforementioned risk constellation, antiplatelet monotherapy is generally sufficient.
b) **False.** In the CASPAR study (clopidogrel and acetylsalicylic acid in bypass surgery for peripheral arterial disease) from 2010, it was shown that infragenual synthetic bypasses benefit from dual antiplatelet therapy, albeit with a slightly increased risk of bleeding. For vein bypasses, no benefit was observed in terms of patency rates, with an equally increased risk of perioperative bleeding complications. However, these were minor bleedings, not severe or revision-requiring complications.

c) **False.** If there are no other indications for oral anticoagulation (e.g., atrial fibrillation or history of pulmonary embolism), oral anticoagulation should not be indicated. According to current studies, compared to antiplatelet agents, it does not improve patency rates after infrainguinal intervention, but does increase the risk of bleeding. Dual antiplatelet therapy with acetylsalicylic acid (100 mg once daily) and clopidogrel (75 mg once daily) for 4–6 weeks post-intervention has proven effective, after which monotherapy with acetylsalicylic acid should be resumed. Prolonging dual antiplatelet therapy does not benefit the intervention outcome and increases the risk of bleeding. Unintentional prolongation (usually simply forgotten and continued without criticism) beyond 6 weeks should be avoided as much as possible.
d) **False.** For so-called high-risk bypasses in the femoropopliteal and -crural segments, oral anticoagulation with NOACs appears to lead to better patency rates than administration of phenprocoumon. However, the current evidence on this question is very limited, with only small retrospective single-center studies available. Nevertheless, the results are significant and quite applicable to clinical practice. Especially in patients who would benefit from NOACs due to reduced responsiveness to phenprocoumon or poor compliance, this can be initiated with a clear conscience based on the available study results.
e) **False.** Administration of clopidogrel 75 mg once daily for 4 weeks after peripheral intervention is carried out "off label" in many hospitals in addition to the VOYAGER regimen. In a subgroup analysis of the VOYAGER-PAD study, no increased risk of bleeding complications was observed, but also no significant benefit in terms of patency rates. However, additional administration of clopidogrel beyond 4 weeks leads to a significantly higher rate of severe bleeding complications and should therefore be avoided.

Question

14. Which statements about the VOYAGER-PAD study are correct?

a) The VOYAGER-PAD study is a multicenter randomized double-blind study.
b) The VOYAGER-PAD study investigates the effect of low-dose rivaroxaban in patients with PAD.
c) The primary combined endpoint of the study was acute ischemia, limb loss, myocardial infarction, stroke, or cardiovascular death.

d) A total of 10,000 patients were enrolled and randomized.
e) Inclusion criteria were age over 70 and symptomatic PAD without prior intervention or surgery.

Answers

a) **Correct.** It is the largest randomized multicenter study with a vascular surgery focus.
b) **Correct.** In the VOYAGER-PAD study, administration of low-dose rivaroxaban (2.5 mg twice daily) was compared with placebo. A total of 6500 patients after surgical or endovascular peripheral vascular intervention were included, evenly distributed between both study arms.
c) **Correct.** The primary combined study endpoint was ipsilateral limb ischemia, limb loss, myocardial infarction, stroke, and death from cardiovascular causes.
d) **False.** The study included over 6000 patients (6564), 3286 in the rivaroxaban group and 3278 in the placebo group.
e) **False.** Inclusion criteria were age over 50 and symptomatic PAD including previous endovascular or surgical therapy.

Question

15. Which statements about walking training are correct?

a) Structured walking training is indicated in every stage of PAD.
b) Walking training is an important component in the treatment of PAD in the stage of intermittent claudication, especially stage IIa according to Fontaine, i.e., > 200 m pain-free walking distance.
c) Walking training should be performed daily for at least 1 h.
d) Walking training leads to strengthening and expansion of collateral circulation.
e) Walking training is inferior to interventional therapy for stenoses or occlusions in the aortoiliac segment.

Answers

a) **False.** Physical activity, especially walking, is not contraindicated due to its positive effects on health and well-being, but is generally recommended. However, it is not a therapeutic measure in the stage of critical limb ischemia (III and IV). Here, invasive interventional and/or surgical procedures are the main focus.

b) **Correct.** Structured walking training, ideally in a group with or without a trainer, leads to improved collateralization and can help avoid surgical and interventional procedures. It also has positive effects on cardiovascular function, blood glucose levels, and body weight.
c) **False.** Current recommendations are 3 times per week for 1 h or 5 times per week for 30 min. More important than the absolute time, however, is that training is performed up to the pain threshold each time. After a short break and reduction of pain, walking should be resumed.
d) **Correct.** Especially in the thigh, with occlusion of the superficial femoral artery, walking training can lead to improved profunda collateralization.
e) **False.** Even in the aortoiliac segment, walking training should still be recommended and performed in stage IIa and possibly IIb according to Fontaine. The CLEVER study (Claudication exercise versus endoluminal revascularisation) from 2011 already showed a clear benefit of walking training compared to intervention, especially in iliac stenoses.

Question

16. Which statements about Prostavasin® (alprostadil) infusion therapy in advanced PAD are correct?

a) Prostavasin® infusion therapy can be administered intravenously and intra-arterially.
b) Prostavasin® should be administered continuously via a perfusor.
c) Prostavasin® should only be given from stage III PAD onwards, not for intermittent claudication.
d) Calcium antagonists, nitroglycerin solutions, and prostaglandins can be administered intra-arterially to prevent peripheral spasms.
e) Headaches, phlebitis, and skin redness at the site of the infused vein are among the most common adverse effects of Prostavasin® infusion therapy.

Answers

a) **Correct.** Prostavasin® infusion therapy can be administered both intravenously and intra-arterially. However, intravenous administration is much more common in clinical practice. Nevertheless, especially during peripheral interventions or in the intensive care unit, the intra-arterial route can also be used.

b) **False.** Prostavasin® is usually administered as a short infusion, rarely continuously via a perfusor. For example, the following regimen has proven effective for intravenous administration:
   1. 2× daily 2 ampoules alprostadil (20 μg each = 40 μg) in 250 ml NaCl over 2 h, duration 10–14 days (depending on symptoms up to 4 weeks).
   2. 1× daily 3 ampoules alprostadil (20 μg each = 60 μg) in 250 ml NaCl over 2 h.

   For intra-arterial administration, the following regimen can be used:
   3. 1 × 1 ampoule alprostadil 20 μg in 50 ml NaCl over 60 min.
c) **False.** Prostavasin® can also be administered in stage IIb and has been shown in studies to improve pain-free walking distance. However, opinions on its effectiveness and usefulness vary widely outside of specialist circles. In the stage of intermittent claudication, it is often administered on an outpatient basis in general practice. The infusion duration should not be less than 1 h. Two hours or longer is better.
d) **Correct.** All three agents cause peripheral vasodilation or lead to spasmolysis. They can be administered intravenously, but also intra-arterially during vascular interventions. The main mechanism of action is a reduction in peripheral resistance, thereby preventing or reducing complications such as spasms, embolizations, or intra-arterial thromboses.
   Nifedipine (Adalat®) 10 mg is preferably administered sublingually. Nitroglycerin solutions fractionated 200 μg as well as prostaglandins (Prostavasin®) 20 μg in 50 ml NaCl 0.9%.
e) **Correct.** Headaches and inflammatory reactions at the site of the infused vein are very common (>1 in 10 treated) complications of Prostavasin® infusion therapy. For this reason, the infusion is generally administered via a central venous catheter (CVC) under inpatient conditions. Other common side effects are hypotension and flushing symptoms. Important contraindications for clinical practice include heart failure, pulmonary edema, chronic obstructive pulmonary disease (COPD), and stroke within the last 6 months.

Question

17. Which statements about bypass materials are correct?

a) The GSV is the preferred graft if the caliber is sufficient.
b) Because of the venous valves, the GSV must always be reversed and sewn in using the "reversed technique".

c) The GSV can also be transplanted allogenically.
d) As autologous arterial grafts, the iliac, femoral, internal thoracic, epigastric, splenic, as well as radial and ulnar arteries can be used.
e) PTFE (polytetrafluoroethylene) prostheses have been available on the market since 1950.

Answers

a) **Correct.** The GSV, with a sufficient diameter of < 3 mm, has the best 5-year patency rates of nearly 90% compared to the alternative of alloplastic bypasses, which, depending on the distal anastomosis, have a 5-year patency rate of 20% (crural) to 60% (supragenual).
b) **False.** Ideally, the vein still has a sufficient caliber distally and can then be anastomosed in reversed technique. If the vein becomes too narrow distally, it can alternatively be used antegrade or in situ. In this case, the valves must be cut with a valvulotome. The vein scissors is a long instrument with a small scissor at the end (available from CM-Instrumente in Tuttlingen).
c) **Correct.** The GSV can also be transplanted as a post-mortem or living donation. Prerequisites are blood group compatibility and immunosuppression of the recipient. In long-term results, fibrosis and aneurysms are often observed.
d) **Correct.** All the arteries listed can in principle be used as autologous grafts. However, their use in peripheral vascular surgery has not become established due to unsatisfactory patency rates and the availability of alloplastic materials with better results. In cardiac surgery, however, they are regularly used due to a lack of alternatives, especially crural arteries and the internal thoracic (mammary) artery.
e) **False.** The first PTFE prosthesis (Teflon®) was implanted in 1960 in a child with aortic coarctation by George Holswade. Since the invention of stretched (extended) ePTFE in 1969, known as Gore Tex®, these prostheses have been increasingly used for so-called alloplastic (artificial) vascular replacement in vascular surgery since 1974. It is made from PTFE powder and lubricant and is stretched at the end of the manufacturing process and coated endoluminally with heparin. Nowadays, heparin-coated prostheses (Propaten®) are preferred, as the risk of graft occlusion is reduced. Interestingly, ePTFE, due to its stretched structure and the resulting microscopic gaps in the material, allows water vapor to pass through, while liquid water is repelled. This is the reason for the so-called breathability of Gore Tex® clothing.

PET (polyethylene terephthalate), also known as Dacron®, is, alongside ePTFE, another frequently used artificial vascular substitute in today's vascular surgery. These are prostheses made from woven or knitted monofilaments, hence the softer and less rigid consistency compared to ePTFE prostheses.

Question

18. Which statements about the epidemiological significance of PAD are correct?

a) PAD is a rare disease.
b) PAD is harmless compared to malignant diseases and easy to treat.
c) PAD has no impact on life expectancy.
d) The significance of PAD for the healthcare system is negligible compared to other chronic diseases (e.g., malignancies, autoimmune diseases).
e) Due to lifestyle changes in industrialized countries, especially increasingly vegetarian/vegan diets and the fitness trend, PAD is becoming less common.

Answers

a) **False.** PAD is a common disease and increases sharply with age. More than 20% of people over 70 in Germany are affected.
b) **False.** Cardiovascular diseases are the most common cause of death and account for more than one third of deaths. Cancer is the second most common cause and accounts for about a quarter of deaths.
c) **False.** Patients with PAD have a significantly reduced remaining life expectancy. The getABI study showed that one in five PAD patients (both symptomatic and asymptomatic) dies within 5 years, compared to only one in eleven patients without PAD.
d) **False.** The costs incurred for the treatment of circulatory system diseases are higher than those for the treatment of cancer or other chronic conditions and are the leading item in the statistics of payer expenditures.
e) **False.** Since PAD is a disease of older age, peaking from age 70 onwards, and the lifestyle changes are primarily practiced by the younger population, there is currently a continuing upward trend in incidence and prevalence. How this will develop in the future remains to be seen.

Question

19. Which statements about best medical treatment are correct?

a) Best medical treatment (BMT) uses three drug groups: antihypertensives, antiplatelet agents, and cholesterol synthesis inhibitors.
b) For pharmacological blood pressure control in patients with PAD, ACE inhibitors, calcium antagonists, and β-blockers are recommended.
c) Muscle pain is a typical and common side effect of statins.
d) There are no treatment options for this common side effect.
e) Evolocumab (Repatha®) can also be recommended initially, especially to improve compliance with walking training.

Answers

a) **Correct.** These three substance groups lead to a significant reduction in cardiovascular complications, especially myocardial infarction, stroke, and limb ischemia including limb loss.
b) **Correct.** ACE inhibitors and calcium antagonists are recommended due to their vasodilatory effect and potential improvement of peripheral circulation, as well as β-blockers (reduction of cardiac output).
c) **Correct.** About 10–30% of patients report muscle pain in connection with statin use, especially with simvastatin and atorvastatin.
d) **False.** Another preparation should first be tried, e.g., from simvastatin to fluvastatin (Cranoc®) or ezetimibe (Ezetrol®). If symptoms persist, administration of the PCSK9 inhibitor evolocumab (Repatha®) is recommended, which in the GAUSS-3 study led to a significantly greater reduction in LDL cholesterol levels and muscle pain side effects.
e) **False.** The preparation, which has been approved for several years, is relatively expensive, so the tolerability of the cheaper statins must first be tested. In case of intolerance, prescription of evolocumab can be justified. It is administered subcutaneously, 140 mg every 14 days or 420 mg monthly.

Question

20. Which statements about sonographic findings of the extremity arteries are correct?

a) Triphasic signals are physiological and argue against a proximal stenosis.
b) Monophasic signals are a typical flow profile in post-stenotic arteries.

c) Biphasic flow profiles are characteristically recorded in stenosis-free vessels of healthy young men.
d) Physiologically, extremity arteries show systolic peak velocities (Vmax) of 50–90 cm/s, which decrease from proximal to distal.
e) For grading stenosis of the SFA, it is sufficient to determine the Vmax in the stenosis.

Answers

a) **Correct.** The physiological flow profile in extremity arteries is triphasic under resting conditions. This results from forward flow during systole, diastolic backflow due to peripheral resistance, and late diastolic forward flow due to the Windkessel function of the aorta. The late diastolic forward flow decreases with increasing distance from the heart, and the peak velocity (Vmax) also decreases. The latter is typically 80–100 cm/s in vessels close to the heart, and only 30–40 cm/s in the periphery at the foot.
b) **Correct.** Typically, monophasic flow profiles occur distal to high-grade stenoses, which is due to reduced arterial inflow. In particular, the pulsatile inflow is absent, so diastolic backflow is regularly abolished. However, this only applies under resting conditions. After physical exertion, a monophasic flow profile physiologically occurs, as this leads to vasodilation in the exercised muscles and thus to a reduction in peripheral resistance. A foot phlegmon can also lead to monophasic flow in the lower leg or foot arteries, even without upstream stenoses. Characteristically, there is a steep systolic rise and a high Vmax of sometimes > 100 cm/s (normal 30–40).
c) **Incorrect.** Biphasic flow profiles are typical in older people, as the elasticity of the vessels decreases over time. As a result, the Windkessel function of the aorta is no longer sufficient to achieve forward arterial flow in late diastole.
d) **Correct.** Systolic Vmax values of 50–90 cm/s are physiological; velocities of > 150 cm/s are typically measured in stenoses, while less than 40 cm/s suggests upstream stenoses. The CFA has physiological Vmax values of up to 130 cm/s, the SFA up to 120, the popliteal artery 100, and the distal popliteal 70; crural arteries are normal at 40–60, and at the foot even just 30 is possible.
e) **Incorrect.** The grading of a stenosis along the SFA is done by determining the ratio of the measured Vmax in the stenosis divided by the post-stenotic value. A ratio of 2 corresponds to approximately a 50% stenosis, a value of 4 to about 75%. The pre-stenotic Vmax is not used, as this depends on

whether relevant collaterals branch off between the measurement site (probe) and the stenosis: before collaterals, the Vmax is higher and the rise steeper (due to lower peripheral resistance) than at a measurement site directly before the stenosis (high resistance). Since the visualization of collaterals and especially their hemodynamic significance is often not reliably possible, the post-stenotic Vmax is used.

Question

21. Which statements about completed studies on PAD are correct?

a) The CASPAR study investigated the effect of dual antiplatelet therapy in peripheral bypass surgery.
b) In the COMPASS study (Cardiovascular Outcomes for People Using Anti-coagulation Strategies), the effect of rivaroxaban 20 mg once daily was compared with acetylsalicylic acid.
c) In the CAPRIE study (clopidogrel versus aspirin in patients at risk of ischaemic events), acetylsalicylic acid and clopidogrel were compared after peripheral bypass surgery.
d) In the TELEX study, the effect of sartans on walking distance in intermittent claudication was investigated.
e) The EUCLID study investigated whether patients with symptomatic PAD benefit from medication with ticagrelor.

Answers

a) **Correct.** In the CASPAR study (**c**lopidogrel and **a**cetyl**s**alicylic acid in bypass surgery for **p**eripheral **ar**terial disease), the effect of dual antiplatelet therapy on the patency rate of infragenual femoropopliteal bypasses was investigated. No significant difference in patency rates was found in the overall analysis, but significantly better results were seen in the subgroup of prosthetic bypasses with comparable bleeding risk. This led to the recommendation of dual antiplatelet therapy for prosthetic bypasses with infragenual anastomosis, especially in cases of poor peripheral runoff.
b) **Incorrect.** In the COMPASS study (Cardiovascular Outcomes for People Using Anti-coagulation Strategies), acetylsalicylic acid monotherapy was compared with the combination of acetylsalicylic acid and rivaroxaban 2.5 mg twice daily. Patients with cardiovascular disease (CAD, PAD, stroke) were included; the primary combined endpoint was cardiovascular events or death. There was a significantly reduced risk of cardiovascular

events with combination therapy, while the risk of major bleeding complications was not increased.

c) **Incorrect.** In the CAPRIE study, patients with cardiovascular disease, i.e., myocardial infarction, stroke, or PAD, were included. Acetylsalicylic acid 325 mg was compared with clopidogrel 75 mg, each once daily. The bleeding risk was comparable, but the rate of cardiovascular events was significantly reduced under clopidogrel (almost 9% fewer events with clopidogrel). In the subgroup analysis, CAD patients did not benefit from clopidogrel medication.
d) **Correct.** The TELEX study is a multicenter randomized study in which the double-blind effect of telmisartan (selective AT1 antagonist) on walking distance in patients with PAD stage II was investigated. Telmisartan is an AT-II receptor antagonist that acts selectively on subtype 1 and thus inhibits angiotensin-II-mediated vasoconstriction. Specifically, this study compared the change in walking distance after 6 months of walking training in patients taking telmisartan versus placebo. There was no significant difference in either the walking distance achieved after 6 min or the absolute treadmill walking distance.
e) **Correct.** In the EUCLID study, patients with symptomatic PAD were included and it was investigated whether ticagrelor 2 × 90 mg resulted in fewer cardiovascular events than clopidogrel 75 mg once daily. The idea and design of the study were fundamentally similar to the ALPHEUS study initiated by cardiologists. In that study, patients with stable CAD were included and the periprocedural complication risk after percutaneous coronary intervention was investigated. In both the EUCLID and ALPHEUS studies, there were no significant differences between ticagrelor and clopidogrel regarding periprocedural complication risk or safety endpoints. The results were surprising, as it was expected that the much more potent ticagrelor would have a significant impact on complication rates.

Question

22. Which statements about ongoing studies on PAD are correct?

a) The BEST-CLI study compares vascular surgical and interventional treatment methods in PAD.
b) The STAR-PAD study investigates the effect of mirabegron (Betmiga®) on PAD in the stage of intermittent claudication.

c) In the MOBILE-IC study (**M**etf**O**rmin **B**enef**I**ts **L**ower **E**xtremities with **I**ntermittent **C**laudication), the effect of metformin on wound healing is investigated.
d) The AGRIPPA study evaluates the effect of weight reduction on the progression of PAD.
e) The background of the PREVENT-HD study is the increased risk of thromboembolic complications in COVID-19 infections.

Answers

a) **Correct.** In the BEST-CLI study (Best endovascular versus best surgical therapy in patients with critical limb-threatening ischemia), the best interventional and the best open surgical therapy were and are being compared, with the primary endpoint being major adverse limb events (MALE), i.e., reinterventions and amputations. In each case, the best current endovascular therapy was compared with the best surgical therapy, with two cohorts: Cohort 1 had an available GSV as graft material, in Cohort 2 no vein was available and prosthetic material had to be used. In Cohort 1, the results after surgical therapy were significantly better; in Cohort 2, there were no differences. However, follow-up is still ongoing.
b) **Correct.** Mirabegron (Betmiga®) is a β3-receptor agonist. β3-adrenoceptors are expressed, among others, in endothelial cells. Stimulation of these receptors leads to increased NO production, thereby stabilizing endothelial function and stimulating angiogenesis. It has already been shown that this can slow down or halt the atherosclerosis process and stimulate collateralization. The STAR-PAD study now aims to investigate the effect of Betmiga® 50 mg once daily, compared with placebo, on the walking distance of patients with PAD stage II. Randomization is double-blind, and recruitment began in 2022.
c) **Incorrect.** The MOBILE-IC study is a single-center study in which patients with intermittent claudication receive either metformin 500 mg twice daily or placebo for 6 months, in a triple-blind design (patient, treating physician, scientist). The primary endpoint is absolute treadmill walking distance under standardized conditions within 6 min. The background of the study is that metformin, in addition to its antidiabetic effect, also has anti-inflammatory properties and apparently can slow down or even halt the atherosclerosis process. Recruitment began in 2022.
d) **Incorrect.** In the AGRIPPA study (**A**pixaban versus Clopido**GR**el on a background of aspirin in patient undergoing Infra**P**o**P**liteal **A**ngioplasty

for critical limb ischemia), the effect of apixaban (Eliquis®) 2.5 mg twice daily together with acetylsalicylic acid is compared with the combination of clopidogrel/acetylsalicylic acid after infrapopliteal angioplasty. Patients with critical limb ischemia without contraindication for oral anticoagulation are included. Primary endpoints are reocclusion or revision after intervention, as well as amputation above the ankle (major adverse limb event, MALE) or a cardiovascular event (major adverse cardiovascular event, MACE).

e) **Correct.** The PREVENT-HD study investigates whether rivaroxaban 10 mg once daily for 35 days in patients with increased thrombosis risk and COVID-19 infection can reduce the risk of thromboembolic complications. However, only outpatients are included; the control group receives placebo. The target sample size is 4000 patients in total, with the primary combined endpoint being venous or arterial thromboembolic events (venous thrombosis, limb occlusion, myocardial infarction, stroke).

Question

23. Which statements about thromboangiitis obliterans (TAO) are correct?

a) Thromboangiitis obliterans (TAO) is a large-vessel vasculitis.
b) TAO affects men in middle age.
c) It is primarily an arterial disease; the venous system is very rarely affected.
d) The first description of the disease was by Felix von Winiwarter in 1908.
e) Absolute nicotine abstinence is one of the most important therapeutic measures.

Answers

a) **Incorrect.** TAO is an inflammatory disease of medium and small arteries and veins, the cause and pathogenesis of which are not fully understood. There is an almost universal association with nicotine abuse. There are some reports of underlying immunological diseases, but these are not conclusive for the etiology.

b) **Incorrect.** TAO primarily affects younger men aged 20–40. Women are much less frequently affected, but there is an increasing number of case reports in women as well.

c) **Incorrect.** In almost half of patients, there is initially venous involvement, particularly superficial thrombophlebitis of the veins in the arms and legs. The deep venous system is extremely rarely affected.
d) **Incorrect.** The first description of the disease was indeed by Felix von Winiwarter (Austrian surgeon), but already in 1879. Leo Bürger (pathologist, surgeon, urologist) later described the histological changes in amputated limbs in more detail from 1908 onwards and detailed the disease in numerous publications.
e) **Correct.** Nicotine abstinence is absolutely essential and can prevent progression of the disease. On the other hand, continued nicotine abuse carries a high risk of limb amputation, often in the form of a major amputation at the level of the lower or even upper thigh. Besides traumatic amputation, TAO is one of the most common causes of major amputation in young patients.

3 Diabetes Mellitus

Question

1. Which statements about the epidemiology of PAD in diabetics are correct?

a) Diabetics make up about 10% of vascular surgery patients.
b) Type II diabetes mellitus is also called "adult-onset diabetes," which is why young diabetics in vascular surgery are almost exclusively type I diabetics.
c) Diabetic polyneuropathy is more common than diabetic angiopathy.
d) About 20% of type I and 40% of type II diabetics develop PAD during their lifetime.
e) About 3–4% of diabetics develop a diabetic foot syndrome during their lifetime.

Answers

a) **Incorrect.** The proportion of diabetics among the average vascular surgery patient population is about 30–50%. Most of these are type II diabetics with a corresponding cardiovascular risk profile. Type I diabetics are much less common, but they do make up a significant proportion of patients with preterminal and terminal renal insufficiency who present for shunt placement.
b) **Incorrect.** Type II diabetes mellitus was formerly considered "adult-onset diabetes" because virtually only patients over the age of 60 developed it. It is usually a diabetes mellitus based on insulin resistance of the target cells. This is primarily caused by obesity, which leads to such saturation of the

S. Regus, *Vascular Surgery: Questions and Answers*,
https://doi.org/10.1007/978-3-662-73387-5_3

target cells (adipose tissue) that the postprandial increase in blood sugar can no longer be converted into fat tissue. However, as the proportion of obese children and adolescents continues to rise, there are now also type II diabetics at a young age, and even in children it is no longer an exception. Consequently, it cannot be said that young diabetics necessarily have type I diabetes. Conversely, there are also increasing numbers of older patients with type I diabetes. They are typically slim and suffer from pancreatic dysfunction, which can be caused, for example, by recurrent pancreatitis, radiation, or autoimmune processes.

c) **Incorrect.** Diabetic angiopathy usually manifests before polyneuropathy, although both are generally combined. Strictly speaking, polyneuropathy is a consequence of microangiopathy, in which damage to the arteries supplying the nerves leads to subsequent nerve dysfunction.
d) **Incorrect.** About one in four (25%) diabetics develop PAD during their lifetime, with type I diabetics being at slightly higher risk than type II diabetics. PAD is understood as the clinical manifestation of micro- and/or macroangiopathy of the extremity arteries and, as in non-diabetics, can be reduced by managing and treating cardiovascular risk factors.
e) **Correct.** About 3–4% of diabetics develop diabetic foot syndrome during their lifetime, with type I diabetics being affected slightly more often (about 4%) than type II diabetics (about 2–3%).

Question

2. Which statements about the classification of diabetic foot lesions are correct?

a) Circulatory disorder in the sense of chronic ischemia is the most common cause of foot ulcers in diabetes mellitus.
b) The classification of diabetic foot syndrome according to Wagner is into stages 0–5.
c) Another classification is according to Armstrong, from A to D.
d) Charcot foot is a typical sequela of diabetic polyneuropathy and is frequently seen in diabetic foot syndrome.
e) Patients with Charcot foot require orthopedic footwear.

Answers

a) **Incorrect.** The most common cause of so-called diabetic foot syndrome is diabetic polyneuropathy. Here, microangiopathy leads to circulatory disorders of the nerves, primarily the sensory fibers. This can result in pressure ulcers that heal poorly and can sometimes lead to very extensive tissue defects.

b) **Correct.** The Wagner classification is based on the extent of ulceration and divides into stages 0–5.
   - 0: no wounds
   - 1: superficial wound to subcutis
   - 2: deeper wound to capsule (one toe)
   - 3: deeper wound to bone (one toe)
   - 4: deep wounds to bone (multiple toes/foot parts)
   - 5: deep wounds to bone (entire foot)

c) **Correct.** The Armstrong classification is from A to D:
   - A: without infection and without ischemia
   - B: with infection
   - C; with ischemia
   - D: with infection and with ischemia

d) **Correct.** Charcot foot, also known as diabetic-neuropathic osteoarthropathy, is a sequela of long-standing diabetes mellitus and is characterized by foot deformity. Due to the lack of pain sensation from polyneuropathy, unnoticed fractures of the bones in the foot occur, with subluxation or dislocation. These are due to the lack of immobilization and rest, which in turn is caused by the loss of sensation. In addition, ulcerations and abscess formation often occur, which may require surgical decompression. The top priority in treating Charcot foot with acute complications is consistent offloading of all foot bones and joints to ensure healing.
   In addition to diabetes mellitus, which is the most common cause of Charcot foot, there are rarer causes such as:
   - alcohol-induced polyneuropathy
   - spinal and spinal cord diseases
   - drug abuse
   - chemotherapy
   - infectious diseases (leprosy, syphilis)

e) **Correct.** In acute Charcot foot, consistent offloading is absolutely necessary, which is usually achieved with an orthosis. Briefly on terminology: an orthosis means the limb is stabilized and immobilized, whereas a prosthesis replaces the limb. The following offloading orthoses are available:

- Total Contact Cast (TCC, plaster cast), molded to the limb and used as a resting or walking cast.
- TCC in two-shell technique, essentially like TCC, but then sawn into two parts and can be applied and stabilized with Velcro fasteners.
- Prefabricated orthoses or frame orthoses, custom-made, e.g., Allgöwer walking apparatus, supported at the patellar ligament, so that the foot is completely suspended and offloaded. On the opposite side, a heel lift is necessary. In addition, it is recommended to wear a compression stocking on the same side to prevent edema.
- Custom-made orthopedic footwear, which should be worn permanently after the acute phase has subsided to achieve offloading in everyday life.

Question

3. Which statements about medial sclerosis in diabetics are correct?

a) Medial sclerosis occurs only in diabetics.
b) Medial sclerosis is also observed in intracerebral arteries.
c) The only difference between medial sclerosis and arteriosclerosis is the affected vessel wall layer (media vs. intima).
d) Calcifications of the lower leg and interdigital arteries visible on plain X-rays are usually medial sclerosis.
e) Vessels altered by medial sclerosis were formerly also called "goose-neck arteries."

Answers

a) **Incorrect.** Medial sclerosis is indeed a typical arterial change first described by the pathologist Johann Georg Mönckeberg (1877–1925) in diabetics. However, it also occurs in other diseases such as renal insufficiency, hyperparathyroidism, or Addison's disease. Genetic causes and a corresponding predisposition are also suspected. However, there is little solid knowledge in this area, and many questions remain unanswered.
b) **Correct.** In most cases, medial sclerosis has also been described in intracerebral, intra-abdominal, renal, and coronary arteries. However, the main location is the medium-sized to small muscular arteries of the lower leg.
c) **Incorrect.** While it is true that medial sclerosis primarily affects the media, whereas classic arteriosclerosis involves changes in the intima, there are

other important differences. For example, fat deposits are extremely rare in medial sclerosis, whereas calcifications occur in both forms. In addition, wall changes in arteriosclerosis are usually shorter, semicircular, and located at bifurcations, whereas medial sclerosis is long-segment and circumferential.

d) **Correct.** Medial sclerosis affects the small and smallest arteries, involving them in a long-segment and circumferential manner. On X-rays, these calcifications are often visible natively, without the use of contrast agents. However, a stenosing process can neither be excluded nor confirmed by this alone.
e) **Correct.** Because medial sclerosis often leads to ring-shaped calcifications of the media, morphological similarities with the trachea of geese have been described. Hence the older term "goose-neck arteries," which goes back to the original describer, Mönckeberg.

Question

4. Which statements about diabetic polyneuropathy (DPN) are correct?

a) In diabetic polyneuropathy, a distinction is made between sensory, motor, and autonomic polyneuropathy.
b) Strictly speaking, diabetic polyneuropathy is a form of diabetic microangiopathy.
c) About one in three diabetics suffers from polyneuropathy.
d) Diabetic polyneuropathy (DPN) is also referred to as restless leg syndrome (RLS).
e) Diabetic polyneuropathy (DPN) is reversible with optimal diabetes management.

Answers

a) **Correct.** Diabetic polyneuropathy (DPN) is divided into sensory, motor, and autonomic types.
   1. **sensory:** Pain sensation is reduced, as are touch and temperature sensation. Clinically, this most often manifests as acral ulcers and pressure points.
   2. **motor:** This leads to impaired muscular innervation and consequently to atrophy of the small foot muscles. This results in deformities such as claw or hammer toes.
   3. **autonomic:** This primarily results in loss of sweat secretion and temperature regulation, which clinically presents as dry and cracked skin.

b) **Correct.** In diabetic microangiopathy, there are typically stenosing processes of small arteries and arterioles as well as capillaries. This leads to perfusion disorders of the supplied organs and tissues. The three most important clinical manifestations are:
   1. the eyes: diabetic retinopathy. Here there is a risk of blindness (amaurosis).
   2. the kidneys: diabetic nephropathy with the risk of renal insufficiency up to the need for dialysis.
   3. the nerves: diabetic polyneuropathy. Clinically, this usually manifests as diabetic foot syndrome.

c) **Correct.** About 30–35% of diabetics develop polyneuropathy, whereas the prevalence in the general population is about 5%. Men are more frequently affected by polyneuropathy than women, and the risk of disease increases with age and duration of diabetes.

d) **Incorrect.** Although RLS and DPN are often diagnosed simultaneously in diabetics, they are two different diseases. RLS is pathophysiologically a neurological disorder due to disturbed dopamine metabolism. It is congenital in many cases, but can also be acquired. However, much remains unclear. In contrast to polyneuropathy (where the gender ratio is reversed), women are more frequently affected by RLS, with a prevalence of 10% in the general population.

e) **Incorrect.** Diabetic polyneuropathy (DPN) is irreversible, although symptoms and associated conditions can often be well managed with conservative measures. These include painkillers (non-opioid analgesics: metamizole, paracetamol; opioid analgesics: tramadol, morphine, oxycodone), anticonvulsants (pregabalin), and antidepressants (mostly tricyclics, preferably amitriptyline).

Question

5. Which statements about amputations in diabetics are correct?

a) Diabetes mellitus is the most common reason for amputations of the lower extremity.

b) 80% of amputations in diabetics would be preventable.

c) Diabetics can obtain a second opinion before any amputation.

d) The greatest risk factor for amputation in diabetics is the availability of physicians in outpatient care.

e) 80% of amputations in diabetics would be preventable through vascular diagnostics.

Answers

a) **Correct.** Of about 60,000 amputations per year in Germany, almost 40,000 are due to diabetic foot syndrome (DFS). Thus, diabetes mellitus is, ahead of PAD, the most common cause of amputations.

b) **Correct.** It is estimated that 4 out of 5 amputations in diabetics could have been prevented with optimized conservative therapy beforehand. This includes, among others:
   - optimized blood sugar control and
   - diabetes management (HbA1c as a long-term value should not be > 7.5%)
   - orthopedic footwear to prevent pressure points
   - wound checks and care

   In patients admitted to vascular surgery for inpatient care of diabetic foot syndrome, the ulcerations are usually already so advanced that amputation (at least a border-zone or minor amputation) is often unavoidable. Especially for infection control in sepsis, this can be a life-saving measure. The goal should therefore be to prevent extensive wounds and gangrene, not to delay or postpone absolutely necessary amputations. After all, one in three diabetics develops foot ulcers or DFS during their lifetime, the development and progression of which are often preventable.

c) **Correct.** In principle, diabetics (and of course non-diabetics as well) can obtain a second opinion on the necessity of amputation and alternative treatment methods before an amputation. This also applies in cases of very extensive findings and manifest or impending sepsis. However, one should ensure that refusal of amputation is signed. In the case of a septic condition and questionable capacity to consent, refusal should be obtained from authorized relatives or a court order for power of attorney should be initiated.

d) **Incorrect.** A prospective clinical study from France published in 2023 found that two factors appear to be decisive risk factors for amputation in diabetics: namely, social status and access to nursing staff. The authors thus highlighted the importance of nursing staff and regular wound checks and care.[1]

[1] Bonnet JB, Nicolet G, Papinaud et al. Effects of social deprivation and healthcare access on major amputation following a diabetic foot ulcer in a French administrative area: Analysis using the French claim data. Diabet Med. 2022;39:e14820.

e) **Incorrect.** It is estimated that about 25% of amputations in diabetics could be prevented by prior vascular diagnostics, especially duplex sonography. In the case of arterial stenoses or occlusions, early interventional or surgical therapy could preserve the limb in one in four diabetics. Since about 30% of diabetics develop DFS during their lifetime and 2–5% of these require amputation, prevention of DFS and its progression is of immense importance for patients, providers, and the healthcare system.

Question

6. Which statements about renal insufficiency in diabetics with PAD are correct?

a) Diabetics with PAD have renal insufficiency in > 50% of cases.
b) Patients with DFS should have close blood sugar monitoring.
c) Diabetic nephropathy is more common in type I than in type II diabetics.
d) Low molecular weight heparins (LMWH) cause kidney tissue damage and are contraindicated in renal insufficiency after bypass surgery.
e) Diabetics with end-stage renal insufficiency should preferably receive a synthetic shunt.

Answers

a) **Correct.** More than half of patients with diabetes mellitus develop diabetic nephropathy, which in many cases receives little clinical attention. This should be particularly considered before administering contrast agents, and careful nephroprotective pre- and post-treatment should be carried out.
b) **Correct.** Patients with DFS due to angiopathy often also have renal insufficiency, which can worsen during infection. Therefore, the administration of oral antidiabetics, such as metformin, should be monitored and ideally temporarily paused. Metformin can accumulate in the stage of renal insufficiency and thus lead to hypoglycemia. The same applies to glibenclamide and glimepiride.
c) **Correct.** Diabetic nephropathy occurs in about 30% of type I diabetics and 20% of type II diabetics. In the PAD patient population, it is estimated that about 60–80% of type I diabetics and slightly more than half of type II diabetics have diabetic nephropathy. This should be particularly considered with regard to any necessary shunt placement, and the veins in the arm should be preserved. Harvesting for bypass reconstruction in the leg should therefore be critically questioned.

d) **Incorrect.** LMWH should indeed be avoided in patients with renal insufficiency, but not because of potential kidney tissue damage, but due to the risk of accumulation with impaired excretion. The main risk is therefore not additional kidney damage, but bleeding complications due to relative overdose.

e) **Incorrect.** Even in diabetics, the native hemodialysis shunt should always be preferred. However, it should be noted that diabetics often also have PAD of the shoulder/arm type, and central stenoses should be ruled out or clarified before shunt placement. In addition, the forearm arteries in the majority of patients with diabetes mellitus show medial sclerosis, so the risk of immediate occlusion (= within 72 h after placement) or early occlusion/insufficient maturation within 4–6 weeks is higher than in non-diabetics. Even in non-diabetics, the Cimino shunt has an early occlusion rate of up to 30%, which should be considered especially in young patients. In older patients with type II diabetes and advanced medial sclerosis of the forearm arteries, a native upper arm shunt is recommended, ideally using the cephalic vein without foreign materials.

Question

7. Which statements regarding perioperative blood glucose management in diabetic patients are correct?

a) Oral antidiabetic medications should be discontinued preoperatively.
b) A typical perioperative complication in diabetic patients is hyperglycemia.
c) Since the patient is usually fasting on the day of surgery, insulin administration should absolutely be avoided.
d) One IU of insulin lowers the blood glucose level by about 50 mg/dl.
e) A perioperative hypoglycemia can be treated with 5–40% glucose solutions.

Answers

a) **Correct.** Oral antidiabetic agents, especially biguanides (e.g., metformin = Glucophage®), should be paused preoperatively for 24–48 h. This is particularly due to the risk of lactic acidosis, which can arise for several reasons:
   1. Inhibition of intestinal glucose absorption
   2. Inhibition of the respiratory chain and thereby
   3. Increase in anaerobic glycolysis

Lactic acidosis is a life-threatening condition. Patients with renal insufficiency are particularly at risk. Therefore, perioperative blood glucose control should preferably be managed with insulin.

b) **Correct.** Due to perioperative stress and the discontinuation of oral antidiabetic agents, hyperglycemia may occur. The danger of hyperglycemia, however, is not merely the elevated blood glucose levels, but the life-threatening hyperosmolar crisis and ketoacidosis. Hypoglycemia is also a typical complication and can quickly lead to loss of consciousness in the patient.
c) **Incorrect.** Although the fasting patient does not consume food preoperatively, blood glucose monitoring should still be performed every 1–2 h. In cases of prolonged fasting or a drop in blood glucose levels, a glucose infusion should be started early and insulin administered. A drop in blood glucose levels during insulin infusion should not lead to a sudden interruption of insulin administration. Otherwise, due to increased lipolysis, there is a risk of ketoacidosis. Therefore, even with low blood glucose levels, it is recommended to continue the glucose infusion while simultaneously administering insulin.
d) **Correct.** One IU of insulin lowers the blood glucose level by approximately 50 mg/dl. However, this only applies when triglyceride levels are within the normal range. With elevated triglyceride levels, insulin efficacy decreases. No more than 4 IU of insulin per hour should be given, even with blood glucose levels > 220 mg/dl. To lower blood glucose levels > 140 mg/dl, 1–4 IU/h are typically administered via a syringe pump.
e) **Correct.** Depending on the patient's volume status, 5–40% glucose solutions can be administered. However, 40% solutions should not be given peripherally, as they can damage the vessel wall. In this case, administration via a central venous catheter is recommended. 1 carbohydrate unit (CU) (=12 g glucose) raises the blood glucose level by about 50 mg/dl. 30 ml of 40% glucose solution (12 g) is a good starting point for treating hypoglycemia both in the hospital and in emergency medicine.

4 Modern Wound Treatment

Question

1. Which statements about wound healing are correct?

a) Wound healing physiologically occurs in three phases.
b) Fresh air must reach the wound, as this allows it to heal fastest.
c) In the case of bacterial colonization of a venous leg ulcer (gaiter ulcer), antibiotic therapy should definitely be indicated.
d) Topical antibiotic therapy should be considered in the case of positive swab results.
e) A wound is considered chronic if it has not healed after 4 months.

Answers

a) **Correct**. The 3 phases of wound healing are

1. the cleansing or exudation phase
   - usually up to day 3
   - Hemostasis, exudation of foreign substances and pathogens
2. the granulation phase
   - lasts approximately until day 7
   - Formation of new tissue
   - Adaptation of wound surfaces
   - Amount of exudate less than in phase 1
3. the epithelialization phase
   - lasts until about day 14
   - Tissue is consolidated

S. Regus, *Vascular Surgery: Questions and Answers*,
https://doi.org/10.1007/978-3-662-73387-5_4

- Exudation is barely or no longer present
- in secondary wound healing, stabilization of scar tissue

b) **Incorrect.** The wound requires a moist environment to heal undisturbed. This is particularly important in the granulation phase and supports the healing process. For this reason, modern wound care emphasizes maintaining a moist wound environment and allowing the wound to rest. This means that dressing changes should not be performed daily, but rather 2–3 times per week, or even less frequently if possible. Daily dressing changes in non-infected wounds during the granulation phase are actually counterproductive.

c) **Incorrect.** Venous leg ulcers, clinically often presenting as gaiter ulcers, usually persist for many months, sometimes even years. Bacterial colonization is almost always detectable, but this alone does not indicate the need for antibiotic therapy. On the contrary, indiscriminate and repeated use of antibiotics increases the risk of resistance development without any benefit for wound healing. In cases of heavily contaminated wounds, treatment with silver-containing wound dressings (e.g., Urgotüll AG®) has proven effective, as these chemically reduce the bacterial load. Additionally, hydrophobic wound dressings can be used (e.g., Cutimed Sorbact®), to which bacteria adhere, resulting in a reduction of bacterial load with each dressing change. However, local and especially systemic signs of infection should prompt antibiotic administration. Before this, abscess formation must be ruled out and, if necessary, treated surgically (debridement, necrectomy, or in extreme cases, amputation).

d) **Incorrect.** The use of antibiotic-containing creams and wound dressings is the exception in vascular surgery. In dermatology, their use is more common, e.g., in impetigo contagiosa in children or other bacterial skin diseases. Here, fusidic acid-containing creams have proven effective. However, increased resistance, especially among staphylococci and streptococci, has been observed. In vascular surgery, limb ischemia is the underlying cause of ulceration, with bacterial colonization or infection considered a secondary complication. Therefore, restoration of arterial perfusion and surgical wound cleaning are the priorities. The use of topical antibiotics should remain an absolute exception.

e) **Incorrect.** A wound is already considered chronic if it has not healed after 4–8 weeks. However, the Initiative for Chronic Wounds (ICW) defines certain wounds as chronic from the outset, including venous leg ulcers in chronic venous insufficiency and ulcers in diabetic foot syndrome. These wounds are considered chronic from the day they occur, as they are associated with underlying diseases that are known to cause significant wound healing disorders and primary healing is virtually excluded. By classifying these wounds as chronic from the beginning, awareness of this issue is raised.

Question

2. Which statements about wound dressings are correct?

a) Commonly used wound dressings include hydrofibers, hydrocolloids, hydrogels, gauze pads, and foam dressings.
b) The foam of the vacuum occlusive dressing (VAC) has antibacterial properties.
c) For highly exuding wounds, superabsorbents are suitable as direct wound dressings as well as secondary dressings.
d) TenderWet® is suitable for non-contaminated, low-exuding wounds.
e) Artificial intelligence (AI) can distinguish between fibrin-covered wound surfaces and wound dressings.

Answers

a) **Correct.** Wound dressings are broadly divided into
   1. fluid-absorbing (hydrofiber, alginates, hydropolymers, PU foam dressings)
   2. fluid-donating (hydrogels, hydrocolloids)
   3. antibacterial (Cutimed sorbact® gauze pads)
   4. sealing (vacuum occlusive dressing)
b) **Incorrect.** The principle of vacuum occlusive therapy (VAC) is the granulation-promoting effect of negative pressure, which is applied continuously or intermittently. The wound sponges used are made of polyurethane (large-pored, black) or polyvinyl alcohol (small-pored, white). The latter can also be placed directly on the skin, e.g., for postoperative, heavily exuding lymphatic fistulas in the groin. The polyurethane foam should only be placed on granulation tissue and not beyond (not even on the skin). The reason for this is the stronger suction effect and thus granulation promotion outside the wound. Antibacterial agents are not contained in the available foams.
c) **Correct.** Superabsorbents consist of a polymer core that can absorb many times its own weight in fluid. Examples of superabsorbents commonly used in clinical practice are Zetuvit® (Hartmann), DracoSuperabsorber® (Draco),

Vliwasorb® (Lohmann & Rauscher), DuraMax® (Smith & Nephew), or Cutimed Sorbion® (BSN Medical). Common sizes are 10×10 cm to 20×40 cm. The superabsorbent consists of a pad containing a white powder (the actual superabsorbent material). This absorbs fluid and turns into a gel from which the fluid is no longer released. A 10×10 cm pad weighs 2 g and can absorb up to 250 ml of secretion.

d) **Incorrect.** TenderWet® are wound pads from Hartmann containing a superabsorbent that, as a special feature, has a rinse-suction function. The wound pads are activated with sterile Ringer's solution before being applied to the wound. Upon contact with the wound surface, this solution is continuously exchanged for wound fluid and germs, as the absorbent's affinity for wound exudate and bacteria is greater. Once all molecules of the wound pad have bound wound components and released Ringer's lactate, the rinsing function ends and a dressing change is indicated. This occurs after 2–3 days. TenderWet® is particularly suitable for the painful cleaning of moderately coated and contaminated wounds. However, these wound dressings do not replace surgical debridement of heavily contaminated or necrotic wounds.

e) **Incorrect.** AI is a very promising and forward-looking innovation in many areas of medicine, including wound care. Especially in wound care, consistent photographic documentation can create an increasingly extensive wound registry. This documents wounds, their healing, and the influence of different wound dressings on the healing process. However, with currently available software programs, it is not yet possible to distinguish between fibrin-covered wounds and modern wound dressings. Therefore, it is extremely important in wound documentation to document the wound after cleaning and after all dressings have been removed.

Question

3. Which statements about causes of postoperative wound healing disorders are correct?

a) The most common cause of postoperative wound healing disorders in the groin is lymphatic fistula.

b) Applying a VAC dressing to the groin wound is only useful in case of complications.

c) The duration of the surgical procedure plays no role in the occurrence of wound healing disorders.

d) Obese patients have wound healing disorders more frequently than slim patients.
e) Wound infections are most commonly caused by gram-positive bacteria.

Answers

a) **Correct.** The most common wound healing disorder in the groin is lymphatic fistula, which occurs due to unnoticed injury to lymphatic vessels and nodes. Especially in repeat procedures, at least every fourth patient experiences impaired wound healing due to lymphatic vessel complications. However, these lymphatic fistulas can often be treated conservatively.
b) **Incorrect.** The term Incision Management System (IMS) refers to the prophylactic, standard application of a VAC seal on surgical wounds. Studies have shown this leads to a reduction in wound healing disorders in the groin and in complications requiring revision. When applied to intact skin, the sponge can remain in place for 7 days. The recommended negative pressure is −125 mmHg.
c) **Incorrect.** Not only the number of previous procedures, but also the duration of the procedure, the amount of blood loss, administration of single-shot antibiotics, use of wound retractors, and choice of suture material all play a role. Tissue-sparing surgery and careful handling of hooks and retractors can help reduce wound healing disorders.
d) **Incorrect.** While the risk of wound healing disorders is higher in obese patients than in those of normal weight, the risk is also increased in very slim or underweight patients. In particular, the frequently observed combination of underweight, nicotine, and alcohol abuse leads to wound healing disorders even more often than obesity. Therefore, in very slim patients, special emphasis should be placed on tissue-sparing surgery, as this can help prevent wound healing disorders to some extent.
e) **Correct.** Gram-positive pathogens are a common cause of postoperative wound infections, especially staphylococci, streptococci, and enterococci. However, gram-negative rods should also be mentioned, particularly E. coli and Klebsiella.

Question

4. Which statements about antibacterial wound dressings are correct?

a) Iodine-containing dressing materials are well-established and should be preferred for infected wounds.
b) The crucial factor in infected wounds is the biofilm produced by bacteria.

c) Hydrophobic wound dressings include Cutimed sorbact®, which has proven effective in infected wounds.
d) Polyhexanide, also known as **P**oly**h**exa**m**ethylen**b**iguanide (PHMB), is a wound antiseptic, but is only approved for wound irrigation.
e) Octenisept® contains high-percentage alcohol and should therefore not be used for wound cleaning.

Answers

a) **Incorrect.** Iodine-containing tampons and wound dressings are still commonly used for infected ulcers, but there are now more tolerable and therefore preferred materials. These include, for example, hydrophobic gauze pads or silver-containing dressings.
b) **Correct.** The biofilm is produced by bacteria and serves as protection against antibacterial measures and substances. The biofilm is the target of silver-containing wound dressings, such as Anticoat® from Smith Nephew. The principle is the continuous release of silver, thereby destroying the bacterial biofilm.
c) **Correct.** Cutimed® Sorbact® is a hydrophobic wound dressing containing the active ingredient **Dia**lkyl**c**arbamoyl**c**hloride (DACC). The characteristic feature of this dressing is that bacteria are attracted and trapped in the mesh of the dressing, where they are effectively immobilized. This is comparable to flies being caught and fixed in a spider's web. Here, too, the hydrophobic effect is crucial. With each dressing change, the bacterial load is demonstrably reduced when using DACC.
d) **Incorrect.** Polyhexanide is most commonly used for wound irrigation (Octenilin®), but is also available as a wound dressing in the form of PHMB-containing foam dressings (e.g., DracoFoam® from Drago™). It very rarely causes local or systemic sensitization or side effects and is well tolerated.
e) **Incorrect.** Octenisept® contains, in addition to the antiseptic octenidine dihydrochloride, 2% phenoxyethanol, but is approved for use on wounds. The manufacturer also states on the Octenisept® bottle that the solution is alcohol-free, as phenoxyethanol is classified as a preservative. The manufacturer only warns against injecting Octenisept® into deep wound cavities and pockets: "To avoid tissue damage, the preparation must not be introduced into deep tissue using a syringe."

Question

5. Which statements about vacuum occlusive dressing therapy are correct?

a) V.A.C.® therapy is abbreviated from the first three letters (**Vac**uum).
b) The silver-containing sponge (GranuFoam silver™) replaces surgical debridement.
c) The "white" sponge can be safely placed on vascular anastomoses.
d) A VAC dressing can be safely applied to closed surgical wounds.
e) The suction for a VAC dressing should always be set to 75–125 mmHg.

Answers

a) **Incorrect.** The abbreviation V.A.C.® stands for **V**acuum **a**ssisted **c**losure and was introduced by the company KCI.
b) **Incorrect.** VAC therapy should never be applied to infected necrotic tissue, regardless of the type or manufacturer of the sponge. Surgical debridement must always be performed first. This therapy is also contraindicated in infected bone processes (osteomyelitis). Careful hemostasis is essential to prevent leakage of the dressing and excessive blood loss.
c) **Incorrect.** The "white" sponge from KCI (WhiteFoam™) is easier to remove from tissue compared to the "black" sponge (GranuFoam™), but should still not be placed directly on anastomoses, nerves, tendons, or ligaments. There is a risk of erosion (anastomoses, blood vessels) and drying out of structures (bradytrophic tissues). Therefore, the manufacturer explicitly recommends placing natural tissue or a non-adherent dressing material (e.g., silicone mesh) between the foam and the aforementioned structures.
d) **Incorrect.** While it is correct that a VAC dressing can be applied to surgical wounds, a non-adherent dressing should be placed between the sponge and the skin, e.g., a silicone mesh dressing, to prevent sticking to the wound.
e) **Incorrect.** Although it is common in clinical practice for the device to be preset to a suction range of 75–125 mmHg, the manufacturer recommends a suction of >125 mmHg–175 mmHg for the "white" sponge (polyvinyl alcohol foam = WhiteFoam®). For the "black" sponge (polyurethane = GranuFoam™), which is widely used in hospitals, a suction of 75–125 mmHg is generally applied and recommended by the manufacturer.

Questions

6. Which statements about debridement and shaving are correct?

a) Debridement of chronic wounds should always be performed surgically using a sharp spoon.
b) Ultrasound-assisted wound cleaning can only be used for non-infected wounds.
c) So-called shaving is used successfully especially for venous leg ulcers.
d) Without the possibility of plastic coverage, no ulcer shaving should be performed.
e) For split-thickness skin grafting (mesh graft), the harvested skin layer should be about 0.2–0.4 mm thick.

Answers

a) **Incorrect.** There are different ways and methods to clean wounds. Certainly, scalpel, scissors, and sharp spoon are part of the usual surgical repertoire and cannot be dispensed with. However, there are now gentler methods to clean chronic wounds and preserve healthy tissue. These include, for example, ultrasound-assisted wound cleaning.
b) **Incorrect.** Ultrasound-assisted wound cleaning can be used for all wounds, especially chronic ones. The device, which resembles an electric toothbrush, uses ultrasound to create bubbles in the irrigation fluid (so-called cavitation bubbles), which remove coatings and especially the biofilm of chronic wounds. Healthy tissue is treated gently and largely preserved. This bubble formation is also called the "cavitation effect" of ultrasound.
c) **Correct.** In venous leg ulcers, dermatoliposclerosis typically develops, i.e., thickening of the skin and superficial skin layers. These thickened skin layers lie on the fascia and resemble it in shape and firmness. With simple debridement using a sharp spoon, these firm and hard tissue layers can only be inadequately removed. Here, shaving is preferred. In principle, superficial layers are gradually removed tangentially until the wound bed is clean and well perfused. Afterwards, a split-thickness skin graft can be applied to these wounds.
d) **Incorrect.** Ulcer shaving can also be performed without plastic coverage, but the healing process is usually prolonged. If too much time elapses between shaving and split-thickness skin grafting (a few days to a few weeks is enough), the wound bed is already covered with a biofilm again and skin graft take is impaired.

e) **Correct.** In split-thickness skin grafting, skin grafts with a thickness of 0.2–0.4 mm are used. Using a dermatome, which can be set to the desired thickness, skin strips are preferably harvested from the ipsilateral thigh. The lateral thigh should be preferred, as the skin here is more resilient and the patient experiences less pain afterwards. A mesh can be created using a roller with slit-shaped blades.

Questions

7. Which statements about cold plasma therapy are correct?

a) Plasma is one of the four states of matter.
b) Cold plasma can only be used for chronic wounds.
c) Cold plasma has a temperature of −80 °C.
d) "Hot" plasma has no application in medicine.
e) Cold plasma is only important for wound treatment in vascular surgery.

Answers

a) **Correct.** There are four states of matter:
   I. solid
   II. liquid
   III. gaseous
   IV. plasma

   Any substance can transition from one state of matter to the next with the input of energy. "Solid" is the state with the lowest energy, "plasma" the highest. 99% of the matter in the universe is plasma, including, among others, the sun.

b) **Incorrect.** Cold plasma is used not only in medicine, but also in agriculture, industry, aerospace, and other fields. In medicine, it is used for disinfection and surface treatment, as well as for surgical incisions and wound regeneration. In wound care, it is particularly indicated for the treatment of chronic wounds, but fresh wounds can also be treated with plasma, for example, to reduce excessive scar formation (keloids). The field in medicine that specializes in the application of plasma is also called plasma medicine.

c) **Incorrect.** Cold plasma has a temperature of 25–45 °C and therefore does not cause tissue damage. Compared to "hot plasma," it is also referred to as non-thermal plasma (NTP). This is because most of the molecules are unstable and maintain the high energy level only briefly, dropping back down within fractions of a second. This creates an electric field, which improves microcirculation. Classic atmospheric plasma has a temperature of > 10,000 °C, as the change of state of matter only occurs at these temperatures.

d) **Incorrect.** Cold plasma (non-thermal plasma) has only been approved as a medical device in medicine since 2013 and has been increasingly used since then. In contrast, hot plasma has been used since 1990, particularly in endoscopic surgery for hemostasis and for performing gastrointestinal and hepatic tumor resections (argon plasma coagulation).
e) **Incorrect.** In vascular surgery, cold plasma is primarily and predominantly used in wound care. However, other areas of application are also noteworthy and very promising. For example, cold plasma is already being used in studies for the pre-treatment of synthetic bypass and stent materials and has delivered very promising results. It has been shown that bypasses pre-treated with cold plasma integrate into tissue more quickly and have fewer complications (such as thrombotic occlusions or infections).

Carotid Stenoses

5

Question

1. Which statements about the historical development of carotid surgery are correct?

a) The first surgical reconstruction of a stenosis of the extracranial internal carotid artery was in 1951.
b) This surgical technique was the standard in carotid surgery for a long time.
c) At the end of the last century, more carotid stenoses were operated on than appendectomies.
d) This trend could be explained by the widespread use and availability of heparin.
e) Only symptomatic patients were operated on, who could increasingly be identified due to improved diagnostic capabilities.

Answers

a) **Correct.** The neurosurgeon Raul Carrea from Buenos Aires operated on a patient with symptomatic carotid stenosis in 1951 by ligating it and anastomosing it to the external carotid artery.
b) **Incorrect.** On August 7, 1953, the cardiac surgeon Michael De Bakey successfully operated on a 53-year-old bus driver who suffered from recurrent TIAs, using the thrombendarterectomy technique still commonly used today, but with direct suture closure without patch plasty.
c) **Correct.** Between 1971 and 1983, the number of surgical procedures on the extracranial internal carotid artery increased almost tenfold (from 12,000 in 1971 to 1,070,000 in 1983).

S. Regus, *Vascular Surgery: Questions and Answers*,
https://doi.org/10.1007/978-3-662-73387-5_5

d) **Incorrect.** Heparin and its anticoagulant effect were already discovered in 1916, after which it became available for clinical use from 1936 and was increasingly used. Rather, the popularity of this procedure (relatively short, operating time approx. 1 h, good revenue) was the reason, not the availability of heparin. Since carotid surgery was being performed almost inflationarily at that time (more frequently than inguinal hernia operations), and given a not insignificant number of perioperative strokes, studies were initiated to determine which patients actually benefit from this procedure, which remains popular among surgeons to this day.

e) **Incorrect.** The indication for carotid procedures was set quite broadly, and both symptomatic and increasingly asymptomatic patients were operated on. This was associated with a rising complication rate (mortality 2.8%!). As a result, randomized multicenter studies (CASANOVA, ACAS, ACT, ACST) compared surgical carotid reconstruction with purely conservative therapy.

Question

2. Which statements about stroke risk are correct?

a) The risk of stroke is lower in embolic origin (atrial fibrillation) than in high-grade stenosis of the internal carotid artery (ICA).

b) In high-grade (> 70%) stenosis of the ICA, the risk of stroke is 10–20% per year.

c) So-called "soft" plaques have a significantly higher risk of stroke than heavily calcified hard plaques.

d) With a contralateral occlusion, the ipsilateral stroke risk in high-grade stenosis is significantly higher than in the absence of stenosis.

e) Men have a higher risk of stroke than women with asymptomatic 60–99% stenoses.

Answers

a) **Incorrect.** The risk of stroke is higher in embolic origin than in that caused by atherosclerotic stenoses. In proportion, 80% of strokes are caused by emboli, whereas only 20% arise from a high-grade upstream stenosis.

b) **Incorrect.** In high-grade asymptomatic carotid stenosis, the risk of suffering a stroke is 1–2% per year. In the large randomized studies (ACAS, asymptomatic carotid atherosclerosis trial; ACST-1, asymptomatic carotid surgery trial), surgical carotid reconstruction was compared with Best

Medical Treatment (BMT). Here, the stroke risk in the BMT group was 10% after 5 years and about 20% after 10 years. However, there was no significant difference between 50–69% and 70–99% stenoses. The study results, however, come from a time when BMT was less effective than today, so it is quite justified to question whether stricter indications for invasive therapy should now be set for patients with asymptomatic stenoses. Especially in patients > 75 years, this should be considered in view of the increasing perioperative risk and the (at least statistically) limited remaining life expectancy.

c) **Correct.** In a 2015 meta-analysis, Gupta et al. showed that echo-lucent, "soft" plaques are associated with an annual stroke risk of up to 5%, whereas echo-rich "hard" plaques have a risk of about 1% per year. However, this fact is not considered in the guidelines of the DGG or ESVS; here, the indication for therapy is mainly based on symptoms and degree of stenosis, not on the nature of the plaques.
d) **Incorrect.** In subgroup analyses of the ACAS and ACST-1 studies, there was no difference in ipsilateral stroke risk with contralateral stenoses in the BMT group after 1, 5, or 10 years.
e) **Correct.** Men have twice the risk of women of suffering a stroke with high-grade ICA stenosis under BMT (1.4–2.8% vs. 0.6–1.4%). This was again shown in subgroup analyses of the ACAS and ACST-1 study results. With the same complication risk after CEA (carotid endarterectomy), men thus benefit from invasive therapy after 5 years, while in women this effect occurs somewhat later (after 10 years) due to the lower risk under conservative therapy.

Question

3. Which statements about neurological symptoms of carotid stenosis are correct?

a) Typical symptoms of high-grade carotid stenosis are dizziness and memory disturbances.
b) A transient ischemic attack (TIA) due to underlying ICA stenosis usually manifests as a contralateral visual disturbance.
c) TIA symptoms, by definition, last < 24 h.
d) The TIA lasts on average 2–3 h and then leads to complete resolution of symptoms.
e) An ipsilateral facial palsy is another typical symptom of TIA.

Answers

a) **Incorrect.** The majority of carotid stenoses are clinically asymptomatic. Hypoperfusion, as seen in the extremities, is almost never observed due to usually sufficient perfusion via the contralateral side and the ipsilateral vertebral artery.
b) **Incorrect.** Most patients with a TIA have symptoms of hemispheric ischemia and movement disorders of the contralateral extremity (usually the upper, rarely the lower), as well as ipsilateral visual disturbances (amaurosis fugax) and speech disturbances if the dominant hemisphere is involved.
c) **Correct.** By definition, a TIA consists of neurological deficits that have completely resolved within 24 h at the latest. TIA must be regarded as a warning sign for an impending stroke; after symptom resolution, there is an increased risk of stroke within 48 h.
d) **Incorrect.** A TIA lasts on average 2–15 min and then has an almost 100% chance of complete resolution. If symptoms persist for 2 h, the chance of full recovery is less than 10%.
e) **Incorrect.** A TIA can cause a central facial palsy if the facial nucleus is affected. However, this manifests contralateral to the affected hemisphere as a drooping corner of the mouth and impairment of the facial muscles.

Question

4. Which statements about speech disorders in symptomatic carotid stenosis are correct?

a) Speech disorders occur in about 10% of acute strokes.
b) Speech disorders fundamentally affect speech production, whereas comprehension is unimpaired.
c) About one in three patients with a stroke suffers from aphasia.
d) The speech center is supplied by the middle cerebral artery.
e) A global speech disorder (motor and sensory) usually indicates a large infarct area.

Answers

a) **Incorrect.** Speech disorders occur in up to 30% of acute strokes when the dominant hemisphere is affected. Due to the predominance of right-handed individuals, this is located on the left side.

b) **Incorrect.** There are different forms and degrees of severity of speech disorders. They are differentiated by severity, type of disorder, and comprehension into

	Severity	Speech production	Comprehension
Global	Very severe	Only single words, no context	Severely impaired
Wernicke	Severe	Often fluent, excessive	Impaired
Broca	Moderate	Single words, "telegram style"	Usually good
Amnestic	Mild	Often circumlocution, substitute words	Unimpaired

c) **Correct.** About 30–40% of patients with cerebral ischemia have speech disorders, of whom, fortunately, more than half fully recover after 6 months.

d) **Correct.** There are ultimately two speech centers, which in > 95% of people are located in the dominant hemisphere in the cerebral cortex. The Broca (speech production = speech motor function) and the Wernicke (speech comprehension) centers. The Broca center is located frontotemporally, the Wernicke center parietotemporally.

e) **Correct.** A global speech disorder with simultaneous impairment of speech comprehension (sensory = Wernicke = parietotemporal) and speech production (motor = Broca = frontotemporal) morphologically and anatomically usually indicates a significantly larger infarct area than isolated deficits. Since the extent of the infarct area can usually only be visualized morphologically after a certain time delay, the severity and quality of speech disorders are important prognostic markers.

Question

5. Which statements about amaurosis fugax are correct?

a) Amaurosis fugax is also referred to as the "TIA of the eye."

b) In amaurosis fugax, patients report a sudden complete loss of vision in one eye.

c) The risk of stroke after amaurosis fugax is 20% within 14 days of the event.

d) Vasculitides can also cause amaurosis fugax.

e) Amaurosis fugax can also occur with stenoses of the brachiocephalic trunk.

Answers

a) **Correct.** Amaurosis fugax is a transient blindness or visual disturbance in one eye, which should always be further investigated. Frequently, there is a stenosis of the supplying extracranial internal carotid artery. The central retinal artery is a branch of the ophthalmic artery, which in turn is a branch (the second after the superior hypophyseal artery).
b) **Incorrect.** After an episode of amaurosis fugax, patients typically report a transient unilateral visual disturbance, usually described as blurred or foggy vision in the affected eye. Complete loss of vision is not typical for amaurosis fugax.
c) **Incorrect.** The risk of cerebral infarction within 15 days after amaurosis fugax is about 5%. However, about 20% of patients already show cerebral ischemia on imaging (usually MRI) after amaurosis fugax. Strictly speaking, these ocular events are then no longer TIAs, but already strokes. Therefore, amaurosis fugax is considered by clinicians to be a serious "harbinger" of stroke, and surgical carotid reconstruction in the presence of underlying stenosis should be performed promptly (as soon as possible within 14 days).
d) **Correct.** Vasculitides can also be causative for amaurosis fugax. In particular, temporal arteritis or polyarteritis nodosa should be mentioned here.
e) **Correct.** Symptoms of amaurosis fugax can also occur with stenoses of the brachiocephalic trunk. However, in these cases, microemboli as seen in stenoses of the internal carotid artery (ICA) are very rare; more often, it is a hemodynamic problem. In this context, it is also referred to as carotid steal syndrome. If the ICA is unremarkable and amaurosis fugax has occurred, it is essential to also assess the aortic arch–proximal cerebral arteries to avoid missing a causative pathology.

Question

6. Which statements about neurological deficits in symptomatic ICA stenosis are correct?

a) In symptomatic carotid stenosis, peripheral hemisymptoms are usually more pronounced in the arm.
b) A left-sided neglect can be a typical sign of symptomatic ICA stenosis.
c) Hemiparesis in symptomatic ICA stenosis is rarely more pronounced in the leg.
d) Gaze deviation is a sign of a severe middle cerebral artery infarct.
e) A drooping corner of the mouth is one of the most common signs of stroke.

Answers

a) **Correct.** In symptomatic extracranial ICA stenosis, an infarct in the middle cerebral artery territory is usually present, and patients develop an arm-predominant paresis or plegia. The difference between paresis and plegia is that in plegia there is complete loss of muscle function, while in paresis there is muscle weakness.

b) **Correct.** Neglect is an attentional disorder and neglect of one side of the body, usually the left. Just as speech disorders can indicate ischemia in the dominant hemisphere, a left-sided neglect suggests ischemia of the non-dominant hemisphere (in right-handed individuals, the right hemisphere). An exact area (center) can rarely be predicted, but it is usually located in the middle cerebral artery territory.

   Note:

   - right (i.e., non-dominant) hemisphere: neglect of the left side of the body
   - left (i.e., dominant) hemisphere: aphasia

c) **Correct.** Since symptomatic ICA stenosis usually leads to ischemia in the middle cerebral artery territory, the resulting hemiparesis predominantly affects the upper extremity. Only if the anterior cerebral artery territory is also or exclusively affected does a paresis of the legs occur. This can also be understood from the homunculus diagram: it is an upside-down little man with oversized body parts (head, tongue, mouth, arms, and hands), which covers the entire middle cerebral artery territory. The legs and feet are thin and small and lie over the anterior cerebral artery territory.

   A complete loss of muscle function, i.e., plegia, is rarely due to cerebral ischemia, but more often due to muscle dysfunction.

d) **Correct.** Gaze deviation is a deviation of gaze toward the hemisphere affected by ischemia, often involving the entire middle cerebral artery territory, especially the anterior parts. The frontal eye field is located here. This unconscious and involuntary deviation of both eyes (without squinting) was first described by the Frenchman Jean Louis Prévost. He also called it déviation conjuguée (Fr. "conjugate deviation"), often referred to as the Prévost sign. In addition to involuntary eye movement, there may also be a turning of the head in the same direction. The déviation conjuguée (in infarction) can be briefly overcome by rapid passive head turning (triggering the vestibulo-ocular reflex). This triggers a vestibulo-ocular reflex. Gaze deviation can also occur with pontine (pons) lesions, but in this case, it cannot be overcome by passive head movement.

e) **Correct.** Since in > 80% of cases, ischemic infarcts involve the middle cerebral artery, the clinical deficits particularly affect the body areas represented and supplied here. These include the mouth (and facial muscles), tongue (slurred speech), and upper extremity. If such symptoms are present, there is a strong suspicion of cerebral ischemia and rapid transport to the nearest hospital is of utmost priority. This is an absolute emergency. This can also be remembered by the acronym FAST (**F**ace-**A**rm-**S**peech-**T**ime).

Question

7. Which statements about staging systems after a stroke are correct?

a) The modified Rankin Scale is divided into 7 stages and describes the degree of disability after a stroke.
b) The National Institutes of Health Stroke Scale (NIHSS) is a scoring system for assessing an acute stroke.
c) The NIHSS score provides guidance for the indication of surgical treatment of symptomatic carotid stenosis.
d) The ABCD2 score is a risk score for the development of a stroke within two days after a TIA.
e) With an ABCD2 score of > 5, the 2-day risk for stroke is > 20%.

Answers

a) **Correct.** The modified Rankin Scale (mRS) is a standardized measure that indicates the degree of disability after a stroke.
   0—no symptoms
   1—no significant disability
   2—slight disability
   3—moderate disability, able to walk without assistance
   4—moderately severe disability, requires help with personal care and walking
   5—severe disability, patient is bedridden
   6—death as a result of stroke
b) **Correct.** The NIHSS score assesses level of consciousness, oculomotor function, function of the facial and limb muscles, facial and peripheral sensation, language, and attention. In total, 13 qualities are scored, with a maximum score of 42 and a minimum of 0. The higher the score, the more pronounced the neurological deficit.

c) **Incorrect.** The NIHSS score provides guidance for the indication of thrombolytic therapy in acute stroke. For a score of 6–22, thrombolysis is recommended; with a lower score, the patient is so mildly affected that, considering the potential risk of complications, they do not benefit from thrombolysis. With a score of > 22, the patient is so severely affected that a large tissue injury, including the risk of hemorrhagic complications or the development of liquefaction necrosis, is to be expected.

d) **Correct.** The ABCD2 score is used to assess the risk of stroke within 48 h after a TIA. The factors assessed are age > 60, blood pressure > 140/90 mmHg, clinical features (i.e., symptoms), duration, and diabetes mellitus. Points are assigned as follows:

Age > 60	No: 0	Yes: 1	
Blood pressure > 140/90 mmHg	No: 0	Yes: 1	
Clinical symptoms	None: 0	Slurred speech: 1	Hemiparesis: 2
Duration of symptoms	< 1 h: 0	> 1 h: 2	
Diabetes mellitus	No: 0	Yes: 1	

e) **Incorrect.** The possible score ranges from 0–7. The risk of stroke is approximately

- with a score of 0–3 = 2%
- 4–5 = 4%
- 6–7 = 8%

Question

8. Which statements regarding the timing of symptomatic carotid stenosis are correct?

a) The size of the infarct area plays no role in the surgical indication for a high-grade symptomatic ICA stenosis.

b) After a TIA, a symptomatic 60% ICA stenosis should be operated on within 48 h.

c) After successful thrombolysis of an acute ICA occlusion with an underlying high-grade stenosis near the origin, surgical reconstruction should be indicated as early as possible within 14 days.

d) A so-called crescendo TIA with underlying extracranial ICA stenosis constitutes an emergency surgical indication; surgical reconstruction should be performed within 24 h.

e) A patient with a so-called “stroke in evolution” should undergo surgery within 24 h, regardless of the degree of ipsilateral ICA stenosis.

Answers

a) **Incorrect.** In addition to the degree of ipsilateral ICA stenosis, neurological status (Rankin stage), and the time interval since the neurological event, the size of the infarct area does indeed play a role in the indication. If the infarct area involves one third (or more) of the middle cerebral artery territory, early surgical intervention should be considered very critically or better scheduled for the interval after rehabilitation. Otherwise, there is a high risk of hemorrhage into the infarct area and liquefaction necrosis, which can significantly worsen the neurological status and the patient will not benefit.

b) **Incorrect.** After a TIA with complete resolution of neurological deficits, surgical treatment of an ipsilateral carotid stenosis should be performed as early as possible **within 14 days**. There is no emergency indication, which is why in most hospitals the operation is performed after 3–5 days and during regular working hours.

c) **Correct.** Similar to symptomatic ICA stenosis without prior thrombolysis, in the case of successful thrombolysis and subsequent unmasking of a high-grade stenosis, surgery should be performed as soon as possible within 14 days. The prerequisite for this early elective procedure is that the neurological status is good (Rankin < 3) and the infarct area involves less than one third of the middle cerebral artery territory. Otherwise, surgery is recommended only after completion of rehabilitation and re-evaluation of the clinical neurological status. At that time, additional intracranial imaging is also recommended to assess the infarct area.

d) **Correct.** Crescendo TIA, characterized by recurrent neurological deficits of increasing severity and intensity, is an emergency indication and should be treated surgically as soon as possible, within 24 h. Thus, crescendo TIA, along with acute symptomatic carotid occlusion, is the most common indication for emergency surgical or interventional therapy.

e) **Incorrect.** Even in “stroke in evolution,” according to guidelines, a pre-existing ICA stenosis should only be surgically treated if it is 50% or greater. In addition, the patient’s clinical condition and the size of the infarct area must be considered: from Rankin 3 or if the infarct area involves > one third of the middle cerebral artery territory, surgery should be postponed and the clinical course observed during rehabilitation.

Question

9. Which statements regarding perioperative anticoagulation or antiplatelet therapy (APT) in carotid stenosis are correct?

a) After CEA for symptomatic ICA stenosis, dual APT is clearly superior to monotherapy with acetylsalicylic acid (ASA).
b) Administration of heparin in therapeutic doses has no role in symptomatic carotid stenosis.
c) Long-term APT with acetylsalicylic acid after surgical carotid reconstruction can significantly reduce strokes in the long term.
d) Brilique® (ticagrelor) is not approved for APT in carotid stenosis.
e) After surgical reconstruction of a symptomatic carotid stenosis, dual APT should be discontinued as soon as possible and replaced by monotherapy with acetylsalicylic acid.

Answers

a) **Incorrect.** According to current studies, after CEA, dual APT does not reduce 30-day mortality (death, stroke) compared to ASA monotherapy. Higher doses (300–1200 mg/day) also provide no benefit, which is why 100 mg ASA daily is recommended.
b) **Incorrect.** Although there is no clear evidence for pre- or perioperative administration of heparin in therapeutic doses in symptomatic ICA stenosis, it is common practice in many hospitals. It is especially used in crescendo TIA, soft plaques, or floating thrombi, and is considered important by many clinicians.
c) **Incorrect.** The risk of stroke in follow-up after surgical carotid reconstruction primarily depends on the result of the surgical reconstruction, but also on the progression of the underlying disease, atherosclerosis. Immediate occlusion is almost always due to technical errors and cannot be prevented by aggressive APT, so urgent surgical revision is indicated. Nevertheless, administration of low-dose acetylsalicylic acid (75–325 mg) is clearly and strongly recommended in the guidelines (Class of recommendation, Cor: I, Level of evidence, Loe: A). However, this is less due to its effect on stenosis of the cerebral arteries, and more due to the significantly reduced risk of cardiac events in the perioperative and long-term course.

d) **Incorrect.** Brilique® (ticagrelor) can be used as an alternative to clopidogrel in symptomatic carotid stenosis. This is especially recommended in non-responders to acetylsalicylic acid and/or clopidogrel. Studies have shown a significantly higher perioperative stroke risk with ASA monotherapy, especially after interventional carotid therapy. Non-responders can be identified with the Multiplate test.
Ticagrelor or prasugrel are P2Y12 inhibitors whose protective effect on cardiovascular events (cardiovascular death, myocardial infarction, and stroke) has been demonstrated in patients after NSTEMI (TRITON-TIMI-38 and PLATO studies). Both, in combination with acetylsalicylic acid, were superior to the combination of clopidogrel and acetylsalicylic acid, but with a significantly higher bleeding risk. Especially older patients aged 75 and above suffered significantly more serious bleeding complications, so the indication should be made with caution.

e) **Correct.** Patients with symptomatic carotid stenosis are usually given dual APT with acetylsalicylic acid and clopidogrel on the stroke unit. This is also the guideline-recommended conservative therapy for moderate to high-grade symptomatic carotid stenosis. After carotid stenting, guidelines recommend continuing dual APT for 4 weeks. This recommendation does not exist after surgical reconstruction, which is why most surgeons recommend permanent monotherapy postoperatively. Since the benefit of dual APT in early elective surgery (with, however, increased bleeding risk) has not been clearly demonstrated, many vascular surgeons prefer to discontinue clopidogrel preoperatively and perform surgery under monotherapy with acetylsalicylic acid.

Question

10. Which statements about vertebrobasilar stenoses and occlusive processes are correct?

a) About half of all strokes affect the so-called "posterior" circulation.
b) The indication for interventional therapy of a vertebral artery stenosis is the same as for an internal carotid artery stenosis.
c) The vertebral artery (VA) is divided into 4 segments (V1–4), with segments V2 and V4 being easily accessible for surgical reconstruction.
d) The prevalence of subclavian steal syndrome in Europe is 20%.
e) In high-grade symptomatic stenoses of the ICA and VA, simultaneous surgical treatment should be indicated.

Answers

a) **Incorrect.** In 80% of acute ischemic strokes, the "anterior circulation" (internal carotid artery, middle and anterior cerebral arteries) is affected. Only 20% affect the "posterior circulation," which is supplied by the vertebral artery. In both circulations, embolic origin accounts for about ¾ of cerebral ischemias, usually caused by cardiac arrhythmias. Atherosclerotic processes and arterial thromboses or thromboembolisms due to stenosis are much less common, accounting for ¼ of middle cerebral artery infarcts.

b) **Incorrect.** The indication for invasive therapy of vertebral artery stenosis is much stricter and more conservative than for extracranial carotid stenosis. This is due to the significantly higher perioperative or periprocedural complication risk. There are only three randomized studies (VIST, VAST, SAMMPRIS) comparing interventional therapy (stenting) with conservative therapy in symptomatic vertebral artery stenosis. These studies and a meta-analysis showed no benefit of stenting over medical therapy. Therefore, routine stenting of symptomatic vertebral artery stenosis is not recommended.

c) **Incorrect.** The vertebral artery is divided into 4 segments:
   - Segment 1 = prevertebral part, from its origin from the subclavian artery to entry into the vertebral canal of the cervical spine
   - Segment 2 = transversarial part, course within the vertebral canal (foramina transversaria C6–2)
   - Segment 3 = atlantic part, after exiting the vertebral canal and passing through the atlas arch to entry through the skull base (foramen magnum)
   - Segment 4 = intracranial part, the intracranial segment up to the union of both vertebral arteries to form the basilar artery

   It is already apparent from this that only segment 1 and a short segment of segment 3 are actually surgically accessible. Due to the high risk of complications, challenging access, and rarity of the condition, surgical interventions on the vertebral artery are rare.

d) **Incorrect.** The prevalence of stenoses in the vertebrobasilar circulation is estimated at about 2–5%. However, this is only an estimate, as most stenoses remain clinically asymptomatic; only 5% develop clinical symptoms. It is correct that about 20–30% of patients with carotid artery stenosis also have corresponding changes in the vertebral arteries.

e) **Incorrect.** The perioperative complication risk with simultaneous treatment of VA and ICA stenoses is significantly higher than with isolated ICA treatment followed by stent angioplasty of the VA. In particular, the risk of perioperative stroke and nerve injuries (accessory nerve palsy, Horner's syndrome) is significantly increased after simultaneous reconstruction of the ICA and VA, reaching up to 30%.

Question

11. Which statements regarding the development of dementia in stenoses of the extracranial internal carotid artery (ICA) are correct?

a) About 50% of patients with vascular dementia and Alzheimer's disease have high-grade ICA stenosis.
b) Cerebral microembolization is considered an important risk factor in the progression of dementia and Alzheimer's disease.
c) There is evidence from studies (Tromso Study) that ICA stenoses (>35%) can already be associated with cognitive and neuropsychological impairments.
d) Buratti et al. published results in 2014 indicating that patients with impaired cerebral perfusion have a higher risk of developing memory disorders.
e) Risk factors for the development of dementia include arterial hypertension, hyperlipidemia, nicotine abuse, diabetes mellitus, and alcohol abuse.

Answers

a) **Incorrect.** In a study by Purandare et al. from 2012 investigating the association between dementia and cerebral microembolization, only 8% of patients with Alzheimer's and 21% of those with dementia had high-grade ICA stenosis.
b) **Correct.** Almost half of all dementia and Alzheimer's patients showed microembolization on cranial MRA, but only 2% had >70% ICA stenosis. However, it was noted that 35% of patients with microemboli had another embolic source (arrhythmia or patent foramen ovale). This underscores the importance of oral anticoagulation but does not justify a more liberal surgical indication in dementia patients with ICA stenosis. This is supported by studies in healthy elderly subjects, in whom asymptomatic cerebral microemboli were detected, but who did not have an increased risk of dementia in follow-up (2.5 years) (Volshaar et al. 2007).
c) **Correct.** In several studies, patients with ICA stenosis were monitored for carotid artery dysfunction and, over up to 15 years, showed significantly more frequent impairments in memory performance and psychological status.

d) **Correct.** The authors found in a 3-year follow-up of patients with sonographically diagnosed high-grade ICA stenosis that those with impaired cerebral perfusion had the highest risk of developing memory disorders and dementia. Interestingly, in patients with bilateral high-grade ICA stenosis but without downstream perfusion impairment, the risk of developing dementia was not increased.
e) **Correct.** Dementia, especially vascular dementia, shares the same risk factors as atherosclerosis. This is evidence for the previously described associations between stenoses of the supra-aortic branches and the dementia syndrome.

Question

12. Which statements regarding anesthesia techniques in carotid surgery are correct?

a) The perioperative stroke risk is significantly lower with regional anesthesia than with general anesthesia.
b) Patients generally prefer regional anesthesia due to fewer side effects.
c) Under general anesthesia, the perioperative risk of myocardial infarction is increased.
d) Cervical block always involves deep infiltration with targeted nerve blockade.
e) The option of regional anesthesia should be offered for carotid surgery procedures.

Answers

a) **False.** The GALA study (General Anesthesia vs Local Anesthesia in carotid endarterectomy) specifically addressed this question and answered it in a multicenter (95 centers in 30 countries) randomized design. Nearly 3500 patients were enrolled between 1999 and 2007 and randomly assigned to surgery under general anesthesia (GA) or regional anesthesia (RA). The 30-day risk of the combined endpoint of stroke, myocardial infarction, or death was comparable in both groups (no significant difference), with 4.8% in GA and 4.5% in RA, and a similarly comparable risk ratio of 0.94 (95% confidence interval 0.70–1.27). Notably, however, there was a relatively high number of intraoperative shunt placements, with 43% in GA vs. 14% in RA. Based on experience, the need for shunt placement in GA with sufficient neuromonitoring is about 1%, which raises critical questions about intraoperative blood flow monitoring and the indication for shunt placement in the study design at that time.

b) **False.** Based on experience, many patients prefer surgery under general anesthesia, as regional anesthesia requires lying still for a longer period with the head reclined, which is uncomfortable for most patients. Additionally, many report a desire not to be aware of the procedure. Interestingly and notably, study results have shown that a previous carotid procedure (usually contralateral) under regional anesthesia was the greatest influencing factor for patients wishing to undergo surgery under general anesthesia. The explanation for this is negative experiences during the previous procedure.

c) **False.** Some studies have reported better cardiac stability during carotid procedures under regional anesthesia. However, none of these studies, including the GALA study (General anesthesia vs loco-regional anesthesia), showed a significant difference in the incidence of myocardial infarction within 30 days postoperatively.

d) **False.** There are three types of cervical block as anesthesia techniques for carotid procedures:
   1. the superficial,
   2. the intermediate, and
   3. the deep cervical block (in clinical practice, this block is usually what is meant by cervical block).
      - ad 1: The superficial cervical block is technically simple and can be performed by either the surgeon or the anesthesiologist. Ultrasound examination is rarely necessary. However, only the superficial layers (cutaneous and subcutaneous) are infiltrated, so intraoperative reinfiltration is always required after skin and subcutaneous tissue preparation. This often leads to delays in the surgical procedure and is also detrimental to patient comfort.
      - ad 2: In the intermediate cervical block, infiltration occurs between the superficial and deep cervical fascia. Spatially, this involves the entire region of the cervical neurovascular sheath, which lies beneath the sternocleidomastoid muscle and above the prevertebral musculature. The use of ultrasound is recommended, and the complication rate is relatively low.
      - ad 3: In the deep cervical block, the local anesthetic is infiltrated directly at the cervical nerve roots in the area of C2 to C4. However, the use of an ultrasound device is absolutely necessary for this. Nevertheless, the complication rate is significantly higher than with superficial and intermediate infiltration. In particular, longer-lasting nerve deficits of the phrenic nerve, vagus nerve, and sympathetic

trunk, which clinically manifest as swallowing disorders or hoarseness, are notable complications.

e) **Correct.** According to current ESVS guidelines (2022), both anesthesia techniques should be offered and routinely mastered, especially the performance of the deep cervical block. The choice of anesthesia technique should take into account the routine and preference of the surgical team as well as the patient's wishes. According to current studies, there is no significant difference in perioperative outcomes between the two anesthesia techniques, although much has changed regarding intraoperative neuromonitoring since the often and solely cited GALA study from 2007. Therefore, a current study addressing this question is overdue, especially given that in the GALA study, the majority of patients underwent general anesthesia without neuromonitoring and with routine placement of an intraluminal shunt. With sufficient neuromonitoring, shunt placement is necessary in at most 5% of operations, which can be explained by the usually adequate collateral supply via the contralateral side and the circle of Willis. Even in cases of high-grade contralateral ICA stenosis (or even occlusion), the need for shunt placement during the clamping phase is low.

Question

13. Which statements about intraoperative neuromonitoring (IONM) during carotid reconstruction are correct?

a) During surgical reconstruction of the internal carotid artery (ICA) under general anesthesia, an intraluminal shunt must be placed.
b) The best neuromonitoring is the awake patient.
c) IONM during carotid reconstruction is based, in simplified terms, on three monitoring principles: functional, hemodynamic, and metabolic.
d) With NIRS, brain tissue can be examined up to a penetration depth of 4 cm using near-infrared radiation.
e) Stimulation of the median nerve during SEP is always performed with the same stimulus current of 10 mA.

Answers

a) **False.** In the vast majority of cases, cerebral perfusion is maintained even during the clamping phase, so only a small percentage require an intraluminal shunt (approx. 3–5%). The indication for this can be determined by various intraoperative measurement methods, e.g., somatosensory evoked potentials (SEP), measurement of brain activity in the electroencephalogram (EEG), transcranial Doppler sonography (TCD), and near-infrared spectroscopy (NIRS). According to currently available evidence, however, there are no contraindications to routine intraluminal shunt placement. The perioperative complication risk does not differ from selective shunt placement under neuromonitoring or in regional anesthesia. Incidentally, intraluminal shunt placement during reconstructive procedures can be billed separately according to the German medical fee schedule (GOÄ), but this should not be a reason for or against its use.

b) **Correct.** Strictly speaking, in awake patients, i.e., during surgery under regional anesthesia, cerebral perfusion disturbances during the clamping phase can be detected most reliably. However, surgery under regional anesthesia has disadvantages, namely that it can become quite uncomfortable and restless in the surgical field. Especially in the event of ischemia, the patient becomes restless, is no longer manageable, and shunt placement can become technically very difficult and prone to complications. For this reason, various methods of monitoring brain perfusion have been developed, summarized under the term intraoperative neuromonitoring (IONM).

c) **Correct.** In IONM, either
   - the **function** of nerve tissue (in EEG and SEP):
     - In EEG, the intrinsic activity (resting activity, spontaneous electrical activity) of brain cells is displayed. The predominant rhythm is alpha (8–13 Hz), measured in 85% of people. There are also beta (13–30 Hz), delta (0.5–4 Hz), theta (4–8 Hz) rhythms, and numerous mixed forms.
     - In SEP, the median nerve is stimulated by surface electrodes, and the resulting action potentials are measured and displayed. In addition, the latency between stimulus and response and the propagation speed of the action potential from its exit from the spinal cord (C7) and the cortical response are shown. Both a prolongation of propagation speed and a decrease in potentials indicate ischemia in the middle cerebral artery territory.
   - the **hemodynamics** (in TCD, transcranial ultrasound), or
   - the **metabolism** of nerve cells (in NIRS, near-infrared spectroscopy) is monitored.

d) **Correct.** With NIRS, oxygenated (oxyhemoglobin) and deoxygenated hemoglobin (deoxyhemoglobin) in nerve cells beneath the skullcap can be measured up to a penetration depth of 4 cm. The sensors applied to the forehead emit light and measure the reflected rays; however, assessment of the middle cerebral artery territory is sometimes limited. In cardiac surgery, NIRS is preferably used to detect hemodynamically induced cerebral oxygenation problems. It has high sensitivity and specificity here, as perfusion of the entire brain territory is of interest. In carotid surgery, its diagnostic value is limited, as the focus is on the middle cerebral artery territory. SEP is preferred here because it more reliably detects cerebral ischemia in the middle cerebral artery territory.

e) **False.** Stimulation of the median nerve must be individualized and is based on the motor threshold. This is determined by the motor response ("thumb twitch," contraction of the opponens pollicis muscle). Stimulation of the median nerve during IONM is performed with a current strength that is 5 mA above the motor threshold. This threshold increases with age. In the average vascular surgery patient (age > 65 years), stimulus currents of about 15–35 mA are used.

Question

14. Which statements about sonographic diagnostics in carotid stenosis are correct?

a) There are different stenosis grading systems in Europe and the United States.
b) Asymptomatic ICA stenoses should be monitored regularly regardless of the degree of stenosis.
c) In sonographic follow-up of high-grade ICA stenoses, the absolute degree of stenosis is more important than plaque progression.
d) With increasing stenosis, the stenosis grades of NASCET and ECST converge.
e) A post-stenotic peak velocity of > 50 cm/s argues against a high-grade upstream ICA stenosis.

Answers

a) **Correct.** In Europe, grading is according to ECST (European Carotid Surgery Trial), in the US according to NASCET (North American Symptomatic Carotid Endarterectomy Trial). The main difference between the two methods is that in the European system, the degree of stenosis is related to the theoretical diameter of the ICA at the level of the stenosis, while in the American system, it is related to the diameter of the internal carotid artery above the stenosis.

In ECST, the theoretical stenosis-free diameter at the level of the stenosis minus the flow lumen is used; in NASCET, the flow lumen at the stenosis is subtracted from the diameter of the ICA above the stenosis. Since the diameter of the ICA above the stenosis is usually smaller than at the level of the stenosis, the calculated degree of stenosis according to NASCET (for the same flow lumen at the stenosis) is always lower than according to ECST. Thus, a 50% stenosis by NASCET corresponds to a 70% stenosis by ECST.

b) **False.** Several factors determine whether regular sonographic follow-up is recommended or not.
   1. **Patient age:** Life expectancy should be more than five years; otherwise, even in the case of a high-grade asymptomatic ICA stenosis, invasive measures would be withheld. A statistical benefit exists only with a remaining life expectancy of > 5 years. Consequently, patients with an estimated life expectancy of < 5 years should not be monitored regularly, even with high-grade ICA stenosis, as there would be no therapeutic consequences. In practice, however, this is rarely implemented consistently, for various reasons, including economic ones, and because it is sometimes difficult to explain this approach to patients and relatives, often leading to uncertainty.
   2. **Degree of stenosis:** The degree of stenosis influences the recommended examination intervals.
      I. For an asymptomatic ICA stenosis < 50%, it is usually sufficient to perform a check every 2–3 years, if at all.
      II. For a moderate stenosis, in addition to best medical treatment, annual follow-up is recommended.
      III. For high- to very high-grade stenosis, follow-up every 3–6 months is recommended, provided that surgical therapy is in principle possible and desired.
   3. **Previous operations:**
      I. After an ICA procedure (open or interventional), sonographic follow-up should be performed. Initially every 3 months; if findings are unremarkable, longer intervals can be adopted.
      II. For recurrent stenoses, follow-up should be at least every 6 months, but again depending on the patient's condition and the general possibility/willingness for a repeat procedure.

c) **False.** The **CARotid Asymptomatic Stenosis** (CARAS) study specifically addresses this question. This is a prospective observational study in which 300 patients with an asymptomatic > 60% (NASCET) stenosis were enrolled in 2020. Sonographic follow-up is a main component of the study, as is documentation of the risk of an ischemic event during conservative therapy. In the 1-year follow-up results, the risk of an ischemic stroke in > 60% stenoses (NASCET) was about 1% per year. However, patients with stenosis progression during the observation period had an almost tenfold higher risk of suffering an ischemic event. Therefore, standardized examination protocols, ideally performed by an experienced examiner under standardized procedures, are extremely important to avoid errors in stenosis grading. There is no recommendation regarding the increase in stenosis grade (as is the case with aortic aneurysms, where an indication for surgery is given for a size increase of more than 5 mm in half a year, regardless of the absolute diameter) for carotid stenoses. Further follow-up results remain to be seen, especially with regard to risk constellation under stenosis progression.

d) **Correct.** In simplified terms, one can remember:
   1. NASCET 50% = ECST 70% (difference 20)
   2. NASCET 70% = ECST 80% (difference 10)
   3. NASCET 90% = ECST 95% (difference 5)
   4. NASCET 99% = ECST 99%

   This is due to the calculation formula:
   - The diameter of the flow lumen at the stenosis is subtracted from the stenosis-free diameter of the ICA above the stenosis (NASCET) or at the level of the stenosis (ECST), and this value is divided by the stenosis-free diameter of the ICA above the stenosis (NASCET) or at the level of the stenosis (ECST). As stenosis increases, the diameter of the flow lumen decreases and both values approach 1 = 100%.
   - Diameter of stenosis-free ICA (free)—diameter at stenosis (stenotic): diameter of stenosis-free ICA (free)
   - free-stenotic/free

e) **False.** Determining the post-stenotic peak velocity is helpful in cases of acoustic shadowing at the level of the stenosis (often with heavy calcification). However, a peak velocity of 50 cm/s indicates a high-grade upstream stenosis (ECST 80%/NASCET 70%), < 30 cm/s indicates a very high-grade upstream stenosis.

Question

15. Which statements about the comparison of carotid stenting (CAS) versus CEA are correct?

a) CAS for asymptomatic carotid stenosis is associated with a higher procedural (30-day) complication risk than surgical treatment with CEA.

b) The non-procedural stroke rate (> 30 days after intervention) is higher with CAS than with CEA.
c) There is a large multicenter randomized controlled trial (RCT) that provides data comparing CAS and CEA in patients with asymptomatic high-grade carotid stenosis.
d) In symptomatic carotid stenosis, surgery has a significantly lower 30-day stroke rate than stent-supported angioplasty.
e) Older patients (>75 years) had a lower 30-day mortality risk after CAS than after CEA, regardless of clinical symptoms (asymptomatic or symptomatic).

Answers

a) **False.** Results from the ACST-2 study, which included more than 3000 patients with > 60% asymptomatic ICA stenosis, show a low perioperative or periprocedural complication risk for both procedures. The procedural stroke rate for both procedures was about 2% and showed no significant differences.
b) **False.** Here too, there was no significant difference in stroke risk between the two procedures, which was about 5% for all strokes and about 2.5% for disabling or fatal strokes.
c) **False.** There are four frequently cited RCTs that compared CAS and CEA in high-grade asymptomatic ICA stenosis, each enrolling > 500 patients. These are:
   I. SPACE-2 (**S**tent **P**rotected **A**ngioplasty of the **C**arotid artery versus **E**ndarterectomy)
   II. ACST-2 (**A**symptomatic **C**arotid **S**urgery **T**rial-2)
   III. ACT-1 (**A**symptomatic **C**arotid **T**rial-1)
   IV. CREST-1 (**C**arotid **R**evascularisation **E**ndarterectomy vs. **S**tenting **T**rial)

   In both individual analyses and meta-analyses of these studies, there was a significantly higher **30-day mortality** (stroke, death each considered separately and in combination) after CAS (approx. 3%) vs. CEA (1.6–2%). The risk of myocardial infarction within 30 days was significantly lower after CAS (0.5%) than after CEA (1%).

   For the **long-term results** (> 30 days up to 10 years), there was no significant difference in stroke rate between the two procedures. The annual stroke risk was about 1% for each. Two additional RCTs with fewer than 500 patients (Lexington and Mannheim) were also included in this long-term analysis.

d) **Correct.** In 4 studies with > 500 enrolled patients (multicenter randomized), results after CAS and CEA in **symptomatic** ICA stenosis were compared.
   I. CREST-1 (Carotid Revascularization versus Stenting Trial)
   II. EVA-3S (Endarterectomy versus Stenting in patients with Symptomatic Severe carotid Stenosis)
   III. ICSS (The International Carotid Stenting Study)
   IV. SPACE-1 (Stent Protected Angioplasty versus Carotid Endarterectomy)

   The 30-day results favored CEA: The risk of stroke, myocardial infarction, or death was almost twice as high after CAS as after CEA (absolute risk (AR) approx. 8% vs. 4%).

   The long-term results, after excluding 30-day mortality, showed no significant differences between the two methods, which applied to both symptomatic and asymptomatic stenoses. The risk of ipsilateral stroke between 31 days and 5 years after both methods (CAS and CEA) was 3%. The annual stroke risk was thus about 0.5 percentage points.

e) **False.** It was assumed that, due to the less invasive nature of the intervention (percutaneous access, no blood loss, no carotid clamping, no general anesthesia, etc.), it would have a lower periprocedural complication risk, but this was not confirmed. On the contrary, subgroup analyses of the four large RCTs cited above (CREST-1, EVA-3S, ICSS, SPACE-1) showed the following for the combined endpoint of stroke and death within 30 days:
   - for CAS, a risk that increased significantly with age (< 60: 3% to > 80: 13%)
   - for CEA, a constant risk without significant differences (approx. 4–6%)
   - in patients > 70, the risk after CAS was significantly higher (> 12%) than after CEA (5–6%)

   Consequently, the ESVS guidelines (version 2023) recommend that patients with symptomatic ICA stenosis requiring treatment should preferably undergo surgery, and intervention should only be considered in exceptional cases (Class I, Level A).

   There were various explanatory approaches for the demonstrated age dependence of CAS complication rates. The authors speculated that access routes in older patients are more frequently calcified and may serve as a source of embolization during the intervention. In addition, with increasing age, changes in the microcirculation of intracerebral vessels are more frequently observed. This may explain a reduced tolerance to microemboli, which occur more frequently during CAS than during surgery. Nevertheless, there are many open questions in this area that are the subject of further research.

Question

16. Which statements about the different techniques of operative carotid reconstructions are correct?

a) Direct closure of the arteriotomy in a carotid endarterectomy (CEA) is associated with a high risk of recurrence.
b) Carotid eversion endarterectomy (EEA) is the technique with the lowest risk of recurrent stenosis.
c) In carotid endarterectomy, a vein patch shows significantly better results than a PTFE patch.
d) In carotid endarterectomy, the longitudinal arteriotomy should extend close to the internal carotid artery (ICA).
e) With a high carotid bifurcation, the digastric muscle can be transected easily with a low complication rate.

Answers

a) **Correct.** Direct closure of a longitudinal arteriotomy after carotid endarterectomy should be avoided, as it is associated with a significantly increased 30-day mortality risk of stroke as well as a high recurrence risk of up to 50% after 5 years. However, the studies comparing direct closure with other techniques are already > 20 years old. This is especially the case because the data clearly speak against this closure technique and it is no longer practiced.
b) **Correct.** According to current studies, EEA has the lowest risk of 30-day mortality and recurrent stenosis over time compared to direct suture and patch angioplasty.
c) **Incorrect.** In comparison to patch angioplasty in the groin region, where an autologous patch can reduce the risk of infection, this plays hardly any role in carotid reconstruction due to the significantly lower infection risk in the neck area. The vein patch in carotid reconstruction shows significantly worse short- and long-term results compared to EEA, as well as to bovine and alloplastic reconstructions. It only performs better compared to direct suture.
d) **Incorrect.** Ideally, the incision for the longitudinal arteriotomy before carotid endarterectomy should maintain a sufficient distance from the ICA

and not extend too close to it. Otherwise, reconstruction can become difficult and associated with a high risk of rebleeding, recurrent stenosis, or immediate occlusion.

e) **Incorrect.** Transection of the digastric muscle in the case of a high carotid bifurcation is indeed a practical option to gain access in such cases, but it carries a not insignificant risk of complications. The main concern is nerve injury, which is why the muscle should be carefully exposed before transection. In addition, the use of electrocautery must be strictly avoided. Three nerves are at risk during mobilization and transection of the digastric muscle:
   I. Hypoglossal nerve
   II. Accessory nerve
   III Glossopharyngeal nerve

Question

17. Which statements about surgical indications for carotid stenoses are correct?

a) A high-grade asymptomatic proximal ICA stenosis should generally be treated surgically.
b) A high-grade symptomatic extracranial ICA stenosis should, regardless of the patient's neurological status, be treated invasively as soon as possible.
c) Elderly and multimorbid patients with a carotid stenosis requiring treatment should preferably be treated interventionally.
d) There are considerations to change the definition of symptomatic carotid stenosis in future guidelines and to extend the time from the index event (currently up to 6 months is considered symptomatic) to 9 months.
e) In the case of acute myocardial infarction requiring cardiac surgery, a symptomatic 50–99% ICA stenosis should always be treated simultaneously.

Answers

a) **Incorrect.** A high-grade ICA stenosis is defined as a stenosis degree of > 60% according to NASCET or > 80% according to ECST. It is indeed correct that, in principle, invasive (surgical or interventional) therapy can be considered for a high-grade proximal ICA stenosis even in the asymptomatic stage, but it should not be recommended uncritically and as a matter of course. Several prerequisites should be met and clarified before invasive therapy. These include:

I. remaining life expectancy > 5 years
II. the perioperative (30-day) stroke rate of the responsible surgeon should be < 3%
III. independent lifestyle
IV. patient's wish present

b) **Incorrect.** In deciding for or against invasive reconstruction of symptomatic carotid stenoses, not only the degree of ICA stenosis but also the patient's condition and the size of any existing stroke areas are decisive. For a neurological status according to the Rankin scale of 0 (no limitations) to 2 (moderate deficits), early operative or interventional reconstruction is recommended. From a Rankin score of 3 or higher, the patient is usually significantly impaired, and invasive therapy should be performed after rehabilitation. Otherwise, there is a high risk of neurological deterioration after carotid reconstruction and subsequent reperfusion of the ischemic area. The latter should not involve more than one third of the affected hemisphere in the case of early elective intervention (within 14 days after the event). For a larger ischemic area, surgery should also be postponed until after rehabilitation. Rankin score and size of the ischemic area usually correlate, so that a high Rankin score generally also indicates a large infarct area.
c) **Incorrect.** Older patients aged 75 years and above with carotid stenoses requiring treatment have an increased periprocedural and long-term risk of stroke after carotid artery stenting (CAS) compared to younger patients, whereas the complication risk after carotid endarterectomy (CEA) is actually lower in older than in younger patients. This has been shown in several randomized multicenter studies (e.g., NASCET, ECST, CREST). Consequently, older patients with high-grade carotid stenosis should especially be advised to undergo surgical therapy. This may contradict the impulse to recommend "less invasive" procedures to older people and must be thoroughly explained to patients and their relatives. A possible cause for the increased procedural (30-day) and non-procedural (> 30-day) complication risk of stent angioplasty in older patients could be increasing kinking of the arteries and reduced elasticity with age. In addition, increasing calcifications in the aortic arch may be responsible for the higher risk of periprocedural embolization.
d) **Incorrect.** On the contrary, there are considerations to shorten the time interval after the index event, which by definition distinguishes symptomatic from asymptomatic carotid stenosis (currently up to 6 months), to 2–3 months. This is increasingly supported by findings and study results

showing that the stroke risk of a high-grade symptomatic carotid stenosis almost returns to that of an asymptomatic stenosis just a few weeks after the index event. Consequently, the indication for invasive carotid desobliteration or intervention will also change and will have to be set more strictly just a few weeks after the index event.

e) **Incorrect.** Before a planned or emergency coronary bypass operation, a symptomatic ICA stenosis should be thoroughly evaluated. Possible approaches are:
   I. simultaneous treatment of both vascular regions by two separate surgical teams
   II. sequential treatment depending on urgency and severity of symptoms
   Since the simultaneous approach is associated with an increased risk of complications, it should be reserved for exceptional cases.

Question

18. Which statements about NASCET and ECST are correct?

a) NASCET stands for North American Symptomatic Carotid Endarterectomy Trial.
b) The NASCET grading is used only for symptomatic stenoses.
c) In NASCET stenosis grading, the degree of local narrowing is related to the lumen of the ICA above the stenosis.
d) ECST stands for European Carotid Surgery Trial.
e) ECST is a grading of carotid stenoses that relates the stenosis to the post-stenotic ICA.

Answers

a) **Correct.** NASCET is the abbreviation for North American Symptomatic Carotid Endarterectomy Trial. Strictly speaking, NASCET refers to several topics:
   I. A study that investigated the benefit of surgical therapy in patients with symptomatic carotid stenoses.
   II. For a stenosis grading of the ICA.
   III. For a group of scientists and surgeons who have worked on carotid stenosis surgery.

b) **Incorrect.** The NASCET classification and stenosis grading does indeed originate from the "North American Symptomatic Carotid Endarterectomy" study, but it has proven itself as a measurement method for all stenoses and has become internationally established. It applies to all stenoses, both symptomatic and asymptomatic.

c) **Correct.** In the NASCET classification, the degree of stenosis in % is determined by relating the extent of the stenosis at the site of narrowing to the ICA above (distal to) the stenosis.
d) **Correct.** ECST is the abbreviation for European Carotid Surgery Trial. This was a multicenter study in Europe, in which just over 3000 patients were included from 1981 to 1994. These were patients with high-grade symptomatic (specific neurological deficits within the last 6 months) carotid stenosis, who were treated either surgically (60%) or conservatively (40%). The follow-up lasted until 1995 and had a median duration of 6 years. It showed an advantage for the surgery group compared to the conservatively treated group for stenoses > 80%. The risk of death or stroke after 3 years was 14.9% in the "surgery group" and 26.5% in the "conservative" group. This corresponded to an absolute risk reduction of 11.6% and a number needed to treat (NNT) of 8.6. According to the results of this study, 9 patients need to be operated on to prevent one stroke.
e) **Incorrect.** The ECST grading is officially no longer used and has been replaced by the NASCET classification. In ECST grading, the degree of stenosis is related to the hypothetical stenosis-free diameter at the level of the stenosis. In the NASCET classification, the relation is to the post-stenotic ICA. The NASCET classification has become internationally established, thus resolving the temporary classification confusion.
In clinical practice, you can remember:
   - a 50% stenosis according to NASCET corresponds to 70% according to ECST
   - 60% NASCET = 80% ECST
   - 70% NASCET = 90% ECST

Question

19. Which statements about the infarct area of a symptomatic ICA stenosis are correct?

a) A critical symptomatic ICA stenosis must be treated invasively as soon as possible, regardless of the presence and extent of an infarct area.
b) In embolic infarcts, those of the middle cerebral artery territory predominate.
c) Hemodynamic infarcts are usually located in the watershed areas.

d) A so-called "lenticular nucleus infarct" is not typical of infarcts due to ICA stenosis.
e) A so-called "malignant MCA infarct" is detectable on CT 24 h after the event.

Answers

a) **Incorrect.** Even a critical ICA stenosis should only be operated on after a recent stroke and imaging evidence of an infarct area if the infarct area involves at most one third of the hemisphere. For larger infarct areas, there is a risk of hemorrhage or liquefaction necrosis and thus further deterioration of clinical symptoms. This is comparable to reperfusion of ischemically altered muscle. Since the size of the infarct area often, but not always, correlates with clinical symptoms, revascularization should only be indicated in a neurologically barely impaired = Rankin 0–2 patient. In a bedridden, incontinent, and non-communicative patient who was previously independent, surgery should be postponed and reevaluated after completion of rehabilitation.
b) **Correct.** The majority of cerebral ischemias caused by ICA stenoses are embolic in nature and most often affect the middle cerebral artery (MCA) territory. Here, a distinction is made between infarcts of the entire MCA territory and those of the anterior, middle, and posterior MCA branch groups. Embolic MCA infarcts do not result from arrhythmias and resulting cardiac emboli, but from emboli that originate in the area of the carotid stenosis.
c) **Correct.** Hemodynamic infarcts do not involve the territories of the supplying arteries (ICA, MCA, and ACA), but rather the "last meadows of vascular supply," also known as watershed infarcts. They are often located in the white matter or extend in a streak from the cortex inward toward the ventricles.
d) **Incorrect.** The "lenticular nucleus infarct," which occurs in the lenticular nucleus next to the lateral ventricles, is also a typical infarct area of a symptomatic ICA stenosis and results from occlusion of the main trunk of the MCA and blockage of the lenticulostriate arteries.
e) **Incorrect.** In a "malignant MCA infarct," which almost exclusively results from complete occlusion of the MCA, cytotoxic edema leads to swelling of the brain tissue and midline shift, which, however, only fully develop and become apparent after 4–5 days. Early signs of a "malignant MCA infarct" are the "dense media sign" and the onset of cerebral edema, visible as

decreased density of brain tissue. The "dense media sign" is caused by the embolus in the MCA, which appears as a dense structure and has a specificity of > 90% for a developing "malignant MCA infarct." In such cases, the indication for surgery should be made with utmost caution.

Question

20. Which statements about recurrent stenoses after operative carotid reconstruction are correct?

a) For asymptomatic recurrent stenoses of the internal carotid artery, the same evidence-based indications for surgical treatment apply as for de novo stenoses (i.e., without prior intervention or surgery).
b) Asymptomatic patients with a recurrent stenosis after stent angioplasty should, according to guidelines, be treated conservatively.
c) For symptomatic recurrent stenoses after carotid surgery, the same indications for reintervention apply as for de novo stenoses.
d) Due to the increased risk of stroke and cranial nerve injury, interventional therapy is recommended for recurrent stenoses after carotid surgery.
e) The risk of a recurrent stenosis > 70% 5 years after operative carotid reconstruction is about 10–20%.

Answers

a) **Incorrect.** The evidence for the treatment of asymptomatic recurrent stenoses after interventional or open carotid procedures is sparse; in the guidelines of the DGG and ESVS, a reintervention is recommended for symptomatic stenoses from 60%, and for asymptomatic ones at the earliest from 70%. Both the recommendation grade (IIb) and the evidence level (B) are, as expected, low.
b) **Correct.** Patients with an asymptomatic recurrent stenosis after stent angioplasty do not benefit from reintervention in studies, so medical therapy, especially consistent blood pressure control and administration of antiplatelet agents, is recommended.
c) **Correct.** Symptomatic recurrent stenoses after operative carotid reconstruction should be treated surgically or interventionally from a stenosis degree of > 50%. This recommendation has the highest recommendation and evidence grade (evidence grade A and recommendation grade I).
d) **Incorrect.** The risk of cranial nerve injury after reintervention is about 6%, but most cranial nerve deficits are reversible. Regarding the risk of

perioperative stroke or death (2–3%), there are no significant differences between interventional and surgical therapy.

e) **Incorrect.** The risk after operative reconstruction is about 4–6%, after stent angioplasty it is 10%.

Question

21. Which statements about surgical steps in the reconstruction of the ICA are correct?

a) The skin incision to expose the carotid bifurcation runs between the suprasternal notch and the earlobe.
b) The platysma should be transected using electrocautery.
c) The common carotid artery (CCA) should be the first vessel to be dissected free.
d) The internal carotid artery should only be dissected proximally to prevent embolization.
e) With a high bifurcation, the digastric muscle can be transected.

Answers

a) **Correct.** To expose the carotid bifurcation, a longitudinal incision in front of the sternocleidomastoid muscle between the suprasternal notch and the earlobe is often chosen. This can be extended proximally and distally depending on the extent of the stenotic process. However, a distance of at least 1–2 cm from the earlobe should be maintained, and if necessary, the incision should be directed behind the earlobe. This can reduce the risk of injury to sensory and motor branches of the facial nerve.
b) **Correct.** Since the platysma has a strong tendency to bleed, it is advisable to transect it using electrocautery. This can reduce bleeding, which would otherwise disrupt the entire operation. This is especially important because, with few exceptions, patients are on anticoagulant medication.
c) **Correct.** The common carotid artery (CCA) is exposed in the lower part of the incision and is located next to or under the sternocleidomastoid muscle. The vagus nerve must be carefully preserved here, and electrocautery should be strictly avoided during dissection. Ideally, after transecting the platysma, no further electrocautery should be used. The internal jugular vein (IJV) lies lateral to the artery, the facial vein drains into the IJV and almost always needs to be ligated and transected. After exposing and looping the CCA and before transecting the facial vein, it is advisable to dissect

the hypoglossal nerve at the upper end of the surgical access. Otherwise, it can be injured and even accidentally transected if it runs deep and gets caught with the crossing veins in the ligatures.

d) **Incorrect.** The ICA must be dissected free to such an extent that it can be easily and completely clamped above the stenotic process. For this, it must be circumferentially exposed. Some surgeons only fully expose the ICA after clamping the CCA and ECA to prevent embolization during dissection and mobilization. However, in the event that a shunt needs to be inserted due to insufficient perfusion via the circle of Willis, this can lead to a stressful situation.

e) **Correct.** With a high bifurcation, the hypoglossal nerve should be sufficiently mobilized, which usually requires ligation of the sternocleidomastoid artery including its accompanying vein. In addition, transection of the digastric muscle can allow further mobilization of the nerve and better visualization in cases of high carotid bifurcation.

Question

22. Which statements about nerve injuries during carotid surgery are correct?

a) The most common nerve injury during operative carotid reconstruction is permanent hypoglossal palsy.

b) In the carotid triangle, 3 neural structures must be preserved during surgical intervention on the carotid artery.

c) Injury to the facial nerve during carotid surgery typically leads to disturbances of the mimetic musculature and elevation of the corner of the mouth.

d) Injury to the superior laryngeal nerve is more common than to the recurrent inferior laryngeal nerve.

e) Injury to the glossopharyngeal nerve is very rare.

Answers

a) **False.** The incidence of nerve lesions following surgery on the extracranial carotid artery is reported to be approximately 5–10%. The hypoglossal nerve is most frequently affected, in 30–50% of cases, although in most instances this is a transient lesion. This can be explained by the mechanism of injury, which most commonly involves lesion or traction from retractors and wound spreaders. Complete transection and thus permanent lesion are extremely rare due to the prominence and thickness of the nerve.

b) **False.** At least eight neural structures must be preserved. These include:
   1. Hypoglossal nerve
   2. Vagus nerve
   3. Recurrent laryngeal nerve
   4. Superior laryngeal nerve
   5. Glossopharyngeal nerve
   6. Accessory nerve
   7. Facial nerve (mandibular branch)
   8. Sympathetic trunk (superior and middle cervical ganglion)

   During dissection, the hypoglossal and vagus nerves are certainly the ones most frequently encountered. However, the other structures listed above can also be injured during dissection in the carotid triangle, resulting in both transient and permanent deficits. The hypoglossal and vagus nerves lie directly in the surgical field and should be deliberately exposed and preserved. The remaining structures are not deliberately exposed if a consistently paravascular dissection technique is used, particularly due to their deeper location. Injury here usually occurs indirectly through electrocoagulation or traction from retractors and wound spreaders. Excessive dissection of the external carotid artery or a high carotid bifurcation are also risk factors for nerve injury.

c) **True.** Mild impairment or restriction of the mimetic musculature is often observed due to transection of the platysma. However, with careful suturing, this is usually only mild, barely noticeable, and transient. If the facial nerve is injured, typically the marginal mandibular branch, there is ipsilateral impairment of mouth corner movement. The nerve is at risk during high cranial dissection in close proximity to the earlobe, as this is where the motor branches exit the stylomastoid foramen. Therefore, it is recommended to maintain a distance of at least 2–3 cm from the earlobe when making the skin incision, and if an extension of the incision toward the center is necessary, to direct the incision dorsally rather than ventrally.

d) **False.** Injury to both nerves during carotid surgery is rare, but injury to the recurrent laryngeal nerve is more common. Clinical symptoms of recurrent laryngeal nerve injury include hoarseness and paralysis of the ipsilateral vocal cord. Injury to the superior laryngeal nerve results only in mild dysphonia, especially with high-pitched sounds (due to loss of the cricothyroid muscle, which as an external laryngeal muscle tenses the vocal cords), as well as supraglottic sensory disturbances, which may manifest as swallowing difficulties, aspiration, and coughing.

e) **True.** Injury to the glossopharyngeal nerve during carotid surgery is very rare and manifests clinically as dysphagia, aspiration, and cough reflex. Since the nerve does not lie directly in the operative field with careful, artery-close dissection, it is rarely injured directly. Here too, injury is most commonly due to electrocoagulation or traction from wound spreaders.

Question

23. Which statements about stents and protection systems in carotid surgery are correct?

a) The risk of peri-interventional stroke can be reduced by protection systems.
b) Protection systems must always be placed distal to the stenosis.
c) Stent design has no influence on the peri-interventional stroke rate.
d) Preoperative "loading" therapy with clopidogrel is only necessary for "open-cell design" stents.
e) Brilique® (ticagrelor) is not approved for platelet aggregation inhibition in carotid stenting.

Answers

a) **True.** In particular, by placing a filter distal to the stenosis, the risk of embolization during the procedure can be avoided.
b) **False.** There are, in simplified terms, three types of protection systems:
   1. Balloon occlusion placed distal to the stenosis (distal balloon occlusion),
   2. Filter protection systems, which are also placed distally,
   3. Proximal balloon occlusion of the common and external carotid arteries (proximal protection).
c) **True.** The two primary differences between carotid stents are "open-cell" and "closed-cell" design. However, studies conducted to date have not shown any significant differences. This applies both to the periprocedural complication rate (immediately after the intervention and up to 30 days thereafter) and to follow-up results.
d) **False.** Loading therapy is indicated regardless of the stent used and significantly reduces the risk of peri-interventional occlusion and stroke. Typically, 300 mg clopidogrel (4 tablets) and 100 mg acetylsalicylic

acid are administered the day before the intervention, followed by 75 mg clopidogrel and 100 mg acetylsalicylic acid once daily from the day of intervention onward. If clopidogrel has already been taken daily for at least 5 days beforehand, loading therapy is unnecessary.

e) **False.** Brilique® (ticagrelor) can be used as an alternative in so-called clopidogrel "non-responders," which should be checked and confirmed pre-interventionally using the Multiplate® test. Here too, a loading dose of 180 mg before the intervention is recommended, followed by 90 mg twice daily on a permanent basis. Although there is evidence of an increased peri-interventional bleeding risk with Brilique®, it is still strongly recommended due to the high risk of stroke with acetylsalicylic acid monotherapy. If heparin is also administered peri-interventionally, the bleeding risk can be reduced by giving protamine.

Question

24. Which statements about stenoses/occlusions of the proximal aortic arch-related supra-aortic branches are correct?

a) Stenoses or occlusions of the common carotid artery (CCA), subclavian artery (SA), and brachiocephalic trunk (BCT) have a lower prevalence than stenoses of the internal carotid artery (ICA).
b) A high-grade stenosis of the proximal CCA should be treated invasively even in the asymptomatic stage.
c) An acute symptomatic occlusion of the ICA with a preceding high-grade stenosis of the CCA at its origin cannot be treated interventionally.
d) A very high-grade asymptomatic ICA stenosis with a preceding proximal CCA stenosis should not be treated percutaneously.
e) There is clear evidence in favor of open treatment of a very high-grade asymptomatic ICA stenosis with a preceding high-grade asymptomatic proximal CCA stenosis.

Answers

a) **True.** The prevalence of ICA stenoses is age-dependent, at <0.5% in those under 50 and >5% in those over 70. Stenoses of the CCA, SA, and BCT are diagnosed in 1–5% of patients with ICA stenoses and have an overall prevalence well below 1%.

b) **False.** Although there is much less scientific data on the treatment of aortic arch-related stenoses and occlusions of supra-aortic branches, current recommendations regarding the management of aortic arch-related CCA stenoses are much more restrictive than for the ICA. Guidelines recommend open or endovascular treatment of the CCA or brachiocephalic trunk only in the symptomatic stage. Due to the significantly increased procedural and non-procedural complication risk, simultaneous treatment of an asymptomatic CCA stenosis during open reconstruction of a high-grade ICA stenosis should be avoided. This also applies to hybrid procedures using retrograde intraoperative stenting.
c) **False.** A very high-grade CCA stenosis with a downstream ICA occlusion can initially be treated radiologically-interventionally without increased stroke risk, followed by intervention on the ICA (thrombectomy, lysis, stent PTA) in the same session. Alternatively, surgical treatment of the ICA with the option of retrograde stenting of the CCA can be performed.
d) **False.** Even with a preceding CCA stenosis (so-called tandem stenoses), CAS can be performed. The CCA stenosis, which in principle does not require treatment in the asymptomatic stage, should or must usually be treated as well. This is essential to gain access to the ICA and is therefore justified. Alternatively, surgical treatment of the ICA alone may be indicated, but in this case without hybrid treatment of the asymptomatic CCA stenosis.
e) **False.** There is no clear evidence for or against surgical treatment based on comparative studies of so-called tandem stenoses of the aortic arch-related CCA and the bifurcation-related ICA. Nevertheless, there is strong reason to assume a higher risk for intervention (CCA with ICA) compared to surgical treatment (ICA only). Consequently, in these rare cases, surgical reconstruction of the carotid bifurcation should be preferred.

Question

25. Which statements about radiation-induced stenoses are correct?

a) Radiation-induced ICA stenoses cannot be distinguished morphologically from atherosclerotic lesions.
b) Radiation-induced ICA stenoses occur in almost one in four patients after irradiation for ENT tumors.
c) Radiation-induced ICA stenoses should be treated like atherosclerotic ones.
d) Radiation-induced ICA stenoses should always be treated interventionally.
e) Radiation-induced stenoses can occur in any irradiated artery.

Answers

a) **False.** Radiation-induced stenoses are typically long-segment and rarely limited to the ICA bifurcation. Since patients often have malignancies of the oral-nasal-pharyngeal region and have undergone irradiation with lymph node dissection, the overlying tissue is often very thin and the vessels lie superficially or directly under the skin. In addition, the skin over radiation-induced stenoses is retracted, which is another morphological difference from atherosclerotic lesions.

b) **True.** The prevalence of radiation-induced stenoses in patients with malignancies of the neck treated with radiotherapy is about 25%. However, since these stenoses are usually asymptomatic, they are rarely diagnosed and rarely present to vascular surgery.

c) **False.** Plaques in radiation-induced ICA stenoses are usually more stable and have a "smoother" surface, so asymptomatic lesions less frequently lead to cerebral ischemia than atherosclerotic plaques. In addition, the perioperative stroke risk is increased in some studies for radiation-induced stenoses. Complications at the access site such as bleeding, rebleeding, and cranial nerve lesions should also not be forgotten. Therefore, many vascular surgeons are much more cautious in indicating invasive therapy for radiation-induced ICA stenoses than for "normal" atherosclerotic lesions. Nevertheless, it should be emphasized that there is no clear evidence for this, so the indication for surgical or interventional therapy of asymptomatic radiation-induced ICA stenoses can also be made equivalently to atherosclerosis.

d) **False.** For a long time, stent angioplasty was considered the treatment of choice for radiation-induced stenoses. However, there is now increasing data on the equivalence of surgical and interventional treatment. In fact, follow-up results suggest that surgical therapy may even be associated with a lower risk of restenosis and fewer re-interventions. The treatment decision should therefore be made individually, taking into account the patient's overall condition, comorbidities, and estimated life expectancy.

e) **True.** Radiation-induced stenoses arise due to an inflammatory reaction in the vessel wall induced and maintained by ionizing radiation. This radiation-induced vasculitis can develop in any artery in the body. However, the carotid arteries are most commonly affected. After irradiation for breast cancer, radiation-induced stenoses of the subclavian artery are sometimes observed, but much less frequently than corresponding lesions in the ICA. Radiation-induced changes in abdominal vessels after irradiation for gastrointestinal or gynecological tumors are even rarer. The key factor in the frequency of radiation-induced ICA stenoses is their superficial location and the resulting increased radiation exposure.

Question

26. Which statements about ongoing studies on extracranial carotid stenoses are correct?

a) The ROCKET-AF is testing whether rivaroxaban 2.5 mg twice daily leads to better follow-up outcomes in patients with carotid stenoses.
b) The CREST-2 study is a three-arm study investigating CEA, CAS, and BMT in symptomatic high-grade carotid stenoses.
c) The CREST-H study compares hemodynamics, especially blood pressure dysregulation, after carotid eversion endarterectomy with patch angioplasty and stent PTA.
d) The ESCALATE study investigates the outcome after surgical carotid reconstruction in patients with crescendo TIA.
e) The "Microembolisation After Carotid Revascularisation" study investigates whether plaque configuration influences cerebral microembolization.

Answers

a) **False.** The ROCKET-AF study is a multicenter study comparing the effect of rivaroxaban at a therapeutic dose (20 mg once daily) with vitamin K antagonists in patients with atrial fibrillation and PAD. In a subgroup analysis, only patients with carotid stenosis are examined. So far, no significant difference has been found between the two anticoagulation regimens, but follow-up is ongoing. In the VOYAGER-PAD study, rivaroxaban 2.5 mg twice daily in addition to antiplatelet therapy was investigated in invasively treated PAD patients regarding limb salvage rate and cardiovascular morbidity and mortality. A significant difference was found, with a clear benefit of rivaroxaban compared to placebo.
b) **False.** The CREST-2 study actually consists of two parallel multicenter randomized studies, comparing CEA with BMT on the one hand and CAS with BMT on the other, regarding stroke risk in asymptomatic patients with high-grade ICA stenoses.
c) **False.** The CREST-H study is a subgroup analysis of patients included in the CREST-2 study who had preoperative cognitive impairment. The aim is to determine whether invasive therapy offers advantages over conservative

therapy and leads to restoration or improvement of memory performance. If so, this could potentially change the indications for invasive therapy in the future, so that not only stroke prevention but also, in selected cases, reduced memory performance could be a reason for invasive carotid revascularization.

d) **False.** The Endarterectomy vs Stenting in Chinese Asymptomatic Carotid Stenosis Patients (ESCALATE) study is a multicenter study in China comparing CEA and CAS in asymptomatic patients with high-grade ICA stenosis.
e) **True.** The "Microembolisation After Carotid Revascularisation" study is a prospective clinical study using diffusion-weighted MRI of the brain to investigate perioperative microembolization risk depending on plaque configuration and composition (soft or hard). Patients with both symptomatic and asymptomatic ICA stenosis, as well as after CEA and CAS, are included. The hope is to gain new insights into plaque configurations that are at risk of embolization with CAS or CEA, in order to favor one of the two procedures in selected cases in the future.

Question

27. Which statements about occlusive processes of the proximal aortic arch-related supra-aortic branches are correct?

a) A high-grade stenosis of the brachiocephalic trunk (BCT) should be treated endovascularly to prevent stroke.
b) The subclavian artery (SA) is the second most common location for stenosing supra-aortic processes after the ICA.
c) Atherosclerosis is a rare cause of subclavian artery (SA) stenoses.
d) A Horner's syndrome can be a sign of subclavian artery (SA) stenosis.
e) If the left subclavian artery is stented over during TEVAR (thoracic endovascular aortic repair), reconstruction of the SA must always be performed.

Answers

a) **False.** An asymptomatic stenosis of the BCT should, regardless of the degree of stenosis, be treated with extreme caution regarding invasive therapy. The situation is different for symptomatic stenoses with embolic complications in the form of cerebral ischemia. Here, urgent therapy is indicated, so **symptomatic** BCT stenoses should ultimately be treated like ICA stenoses.
b) **False.** The SA is the third most common site, after the ICA and vertebral arteries, to be affected by stenosing processes. It is often seen only as an incidental finding during further evaluation of carotid stenoses. The

prevalence in the general population is about 1–2%, and in patients with known atherosclerosis >10%. The left side is more frequently affected than the right, possibly due to a steeper vessel course and resulting turbulence.

c) **False.** Atherosclerosis also plays the most significant role in the etiology of stenoses in the SA. However, in this vascular area, other causes such as thoracic outlet syndrome, inflammatory diseases like Takayasu arteritis, giant cell arteritis, or syphilis, as well as kinking stenoses, congenital vascular anomalies, or fibromuscular dysplasia, must also be considered.
d) **True.** Horner's syndrome is characterized by ptosis, miosis, and enophthalmos. It can be the first clinical sign of vertebrobasilar insufficiency. The cause is hypoperfusion of the medulla oblongata, with stenoses or occlusions of the vertebral or basilar arteries in particular leading to ischemia of the posterior circulation, including the medulla oblongata. This ischemia in the posterior circulation can present clinically in various ways. According to the original describer, this is also called Wallenberg syndrome; characteristic symptoms include, ipsilaterally, in addition to Horner's syndrome, nystagmus, diminished corneal reflex, facial sensory disturbance, vocal cord paralysis, palatal paresis, and hemiataxia. Contralaterally, there may be dissociated sensory disturbance, i.e., impaired temperature and pain sensation with preserved touch sensation, throughout the body. A tendency to fall toward the affected side is also typical.
e) **False.** There is no clear evidence that the left SA must always be reconstructed if it is intentionally or unintentionally stented over during TEVAR. The 2017 ESVS guidelines recommend reconstruction if the patient is at high risk of developing neurological problems. However, the recommendation grade is low due to insufficient evidence (recommendation grade IIA, evidence level C). If there is a left-dominant vertebral artery or a left-sided internal thoracic artery bypass, revascularization is recommended both in emergency and elective settings. The recommendation grade is high, but the evidence level is also low (recommendation grade I, evidence level C).

Question

28. Which statements about completed multicenter RCT studies of the carotid arteries are correct?

a) The SPACE study compared CAS with CEA in asymptomatic carotid stenoses.
b) The SPACE-2 study compared CAS and CEA in asymptomatic ICA stenoses.

c) The NASCET and ECST studies demonstrated the superiority of CEA in symptomatic ICA stenoses.
d) The ACST-1 study (asymptomatic carotid surgery trial) compared CEA with conservative therapy in high-grade asymptomatic ICA stenoses.
e) The ACST-2 study compared CEA+BMT vs. BMT alone in symptomatic ICA stenoses.

Answers

a) **False.** In the SPACE study (Stent-protected Percutaneous Angioplasty of the Carotid versus Endarterectomy), patients with high-grade symptomatic ICA stenoses were included. The criterion was a stenosis of more than 70% (according to ECST) or 50% according to NASCET, as well as a neurological event ipsilateral within less than 180 days. Surgical and interventional therapies were compared. The primary endpoints were death and stroke within 30 days postoperatively. No significant difference was found; the complication rate was below 4% in both groups.
b) **Correct.** In the recruitment phase of the SPACE-2 study, which began in 2008, CAS+BMT and CEA+BMT were compared with BMT alone. Patients with high-grade asymptomatic ICA stenoses were included. However, the study was discontinued in 2015 due to insufficient patient recruitment.
c) **False.** In both the NASCET (United States) and ECST (Europe) studies, it was shown that CEA was superior to purely conservative therapy (BMT) in asymptomatic high-grade ICA stenoses. The studies date from 1993 (and following years).
d) **Correct.** In the ACST-1 study, CEA+BMT was compared with BMT alone in high-grade asymptomatic ICA stenoses. A significant reduction in stroke risk after CEA was observed in the follow-up, which continued for more than 10 years.
   Other studies that compared CEA with conservative therapy in asymptomatic ICA stenoses were
   - ACAS trial from 1995 (asymptomatic carotid artery surgery),
   - VA trial from 1993 (Veterans Affairs)

   and for symptomatic ICA stenoses, these were
   - NASCET and
   - ECST.
e) **False.** In the ACST-2 study (asymptomatic carotid surgery trial), CEA was compared with CAS (each including BMT) in high-grade asymptomatic ICA stenoses. In the follow-up of over 12 years, no significant difference in stroke rate was observed between the two treatment modalities.

Question

29. Which statements about the carotid body (Glomus caroticum) are correct?

a) The carotid body consists of chemoreceptors.
b) The carotid body is a sympathetic ganglion.
c) Carotid body tumors are malignant neoplasms arising from the vessel wall.
d) The carotid body is regularly visible macroscopically during carotid TEA.
e) The carotid body is regularly injured and denervated during carotid EEA.

Answers

a) **Correct.** The carotid body is an area about 3 mm in diameter at the carotid bifurcation and contains chemoreceptors that measure the partial pressure of oxygen and carbon dioxide as well as the pH value of the blood. Glomus (Latin = ball) and caroticum (from the Greek: kara = head). This regulates the circulatory and respiratory centers in the medulla oblongata.
b) **False.** The carotid body is a paraganglion (a collection of autonomic nerve cells) with parasympathetic cells. It is non-chromaffin (in contrast to the chromaffin sympathetic paraganglia) and regulates the circulatory system via chemo- and baroreceptors. Manipulation of the carotid body during carotid surgery often leads to drops in blood pressure or asystole, as the circulatory center in the medulla oblongata is "tricked" into perceiving an excessively high blood pressure.
c) **False.** Carotid body tumors are usually benign, neuroendocrine tumors, which actually have nothing to do with the field of vascular surgery. Overlap occurs only due to their immediate proximity to the carotid bifurcation, often necessitating reconstruction of the carotid bifurcation.
d) **False.** The carotid body is not visible, but manipulations are clearly noticeable due to marked dysregulation of the circulatory system. It is usually located directly at the bifurcation, sometimes also at the bulb of the CCA.
e) **Correct.** During carotid reconstruction, partial injury and denervation of the carotid body regularly occur, which can lead to transient blood pressure dysregulation intra- and postoperatively. This appears to occur more frequently during EEA, but there is no clear evidence for this.

Aneurysms

6

Question

1. Which statements regarding the definition of an aneurysm are correct?

a) By definition, an aneurysm is a bulging of the entire vessel wall.
b) An aneurysm is defined as a dilation of at least 1.5 times the diameter of the adjacent normal vessel.
c) A false aneurysm is, strictly speaking, a pulsating hematoma.
d) An aneurysma dissecans is an aneurysm that arises due to a dissection.
e) The so-called mycotic aneurysm is caused by fungi.

Answers

a) **Incorrect.** By definition, it is a bulging (from ancient Greek ἀνεύρυσμα *aneúrysma* 'dilation, expansion'). In a true aneurysm, the entire vessel wall, i.e., all three layers, is involved. In a false aneurysm, there is a local discontinuity (usually iatrogenic after puncture) and the formation of a perivascular pulsating hematoma.
b) **Correct.** An aneurysm is defined as a diameter more than 1.5 times that of the adjacent normal vessel; the transition from a normal vessel to an aneurysm is also referred to as ectasia. However, there is no exact definition of when ectasia begins.
c) **Correct.** Aneurysms are classified as true and false, a distinction that dates back to before the introduction of sonography. False aneurysms were already described during World War I, mostly caused by gunshot wounds. Clinically, they presented as pulsating swellings and could thus be

S. Regus, *Vascular Surgery: Questions and Answers*,
https://doi.org/10.1007/978-3-662-73387-5_6

attributed to the vascular system. Only from around 1970 was ultrasound introduced and increasingly used in clinical practice, leading to the distinction between true (bulging of the entire vessel wall) and false (pulsating hematoma due to vessel wall injury) aneurysms.

d) **Incorrect.** An aneurysma dissecans is a simultaneous bulging and tear of the vessel wall, usually in the area of the aorta. When diagnosing an aneurysma dissecans, it is not clear which came first: the dissection or the aneurysm. Both are possible:
   I. first the tear in the vessel wall, followed by bulging due to loss of elasticity, or
   II. first the bulging, then the tear due to increasing stretching of the arterial wall.

   For further therapy, however, this is not decisive; rather, the location of the dissection (keyword Stanford A and B), the diameter, and the clinical symptoms are more important.
e) **Incorrect.** In general, a mycotic aneurysm is synonymous with an infected aneurysm. It accounts for about 1–3% of aneurysms and can be caused by any pathogens and infectious agents. However, bacteria are most commonly responsible; fungi are only rarely involved. Pathogens include Brucella, Staphylococcus aureus, Salmonella, Chlamydia, Mycobacteria, and also Treponema pallidum. The term "mycotic aneurysm" was coined by William Osler (a Canadian physician), who chose it because mycotic aortic aneurysms appeared morphologically (intraoperatively) like a fungus.

Question

2. Which statements regarding the distinction between true and false aneurysms are correct?

a) A false aneurysm has a diameter of < 3 cm and is therefore called "false."
b) A false aneurysm can be congenital or acquired.
c) True aneurysms are more common in clinical practice than false ones.
d) False aneurysms are classified pathomorphologically as dissections.
e) True aneurysms are defined by their maximum diameter.

Answers

a) **Incorrect.** A false aneurysm is called "false" because there is no bulging of all wall layers. Rather, a defect in the vessel wall leads to a perivascular hematoma, which subsequently becomes encapsulated. Therefore, the more accurate term would be "pulsating hematoma" instead of aneurysm. The terminology is historical and dates back to before the advent of ultrasound diagnostics. Unlike true aneurysms, there is no diameter criterion for defining a false aneurysm; it is independent of size and diameter.

b) **Incorrect.** A false aneurysm is always acquired and can result from various causes and interventions. Most commonly, it is observed in the groin after percutaneous access, usually during angiography. Inflammatory processes can also be responsible, e.g., false aneurysms in the visceral arteries due to chronic pancreatitis. Traumatic causes, though rare, are also noteworthy, such as a false aneurysm of the profunda femoris artery in the context of a proximal femoral fracture.
c) **Incorrect.** The most common aneurysm in clinical practice is the false aneurysm in the groin after puncture during angiography. However, most of these aneurysms can be managed conservatively and are therefore not referred to vascular surgery. Additionally, the increase in radial punctures for coronary angiography and intervention has led to a reduction in false, iatrogenic aneurysms. This trend is expected to continue.
d) **Incorrect.** Dissections involve a tear in the vessel wall without perforation to the outside. This leads to a dissection, i.e., a separation of the wall layers, usually starting from the media layer. This must be distinguished from an aneurysma dissecans, which is not a false aneurysm but a true one. In addition to bulging of all wall layers, there is also a tear in the vessel wall, again without perforation to the outside. If there is perforation to the outside, it is, by definition, a ruptured aneurysma dissecans, not a false aneurysm (aneurysma spurium).
e) **Correct.** For true aneurysms, the maximum diameter, unlike in false aneurysms, plays a role in the definition. An aneurysm is defined as a diameter 1.5 times that of the healthy adjacent vessel; below that, it is called ectasia. However, this classification and definition are too complicated or impractical for clinical practice, so international consensus has been reached on certain threshold values. The most common value is for AAA: here, an aneurysm is defined as ≥ 3 cm, and 2–3 cm is considered ectasia. Interestingly, the physiological diameter of the abdominal aorta is 1.9 cm in men and 1.6 cm in women. Thus, strictly speaking, an aneurysm should be diagnosed at 2.9 cm in men and 2.5 cm in women. However, this has not become standard in clinical practice. It should be noted that although women develop AAA much less frequently than men, an aneurysm should be diagnosed at a smaller diameter in women, and their risk of rupture is higher. Therefore, according to guidelines, the indication for invasive

aneurysm exclusion in women should be made more liberally at a maximum diameter of 5 cm.

Question

3. Which statements regarding risk factors for the development of an aortic aneurysm are correct?

a) Nicotine abuse is one of the most significant risk factors for the development of an aortic aneurysm.
b) Diabetes mellitus is, after smoking, the most important risk factor for the development and progression of aortic aneurysms.
c) The number of cigarettes smoked has no influence on the risk of developing an aortic aneurysm.
d) Women now have a risk of developing an aortic aneurysm similar to that of men.
e) Since women have a significantly lower risk of developing an aortic aneurysm than men, screening is generally not necessary for women.

Answers

a) **Correct.** Smoking is one of the most important risk factors for the development and progression of an aortic aneurysm. Nicotine appears to play a particular role in the pathogenesis of atherosclerotic processes in the aortoiliac vascular segment, less so in the peripheral segment. This is evident in clinical practice by the distribution and location of stenoses and occlusions (smokers more centrally, diabetics more peripherally). The exact reasons for the preference of the aortoiliac tract for nicotine are unknown.
b) **Incorrect.** Diabetes mellitus appears in some studies to even have a protective effect, which is currently being investigated in detail. It is suspected that metformin may reduce the growth and rupture rate of abdominal aortic aneurysms.
c) **Incorrect.** The risk increases with the number of cigarettes smoked per day; with 5 cigarettes, it is about twice as high as in non-smokers, with 10 it increases threefold, and with 25 it is about 6–8 times higher. On the other hand, the risk for a former smoker who has abstained from nicotine for 25 years approaches that of a non-smoker. However, even after 10 years of abstinence, the risk remains significantly elevated.
d) **Incorrect.** Men are significantly more frequently affected than women, even though the gender ratio has narrowed somewhat. Currently, it is about

5:1. About 3% of men and 0.5% of women develop an aortic aneurysm during their lifetime. This already takes into account different size thresholds: 5.5 cm maximum diameter for men, 5.0 cm for women.

e) **Incorrect.** Although screening is recommended for men from age 65, this is not generally established or included in guidelines for women. Nevertheless, women with risk factors—including nicotine abuse, arterial hypertension, and a family history—should be included in screening programs. Therefore, it is not correct to consider screening unnecessary for women from the outset. Women with risk factors should also receive a screening examination by age 65 at the latest. In this context, it is advisable to develop a certain sensitivity regarding the different treatment of men and women with vascular diseases. Women are still significantly underserved, have an increased risk of rupture, and a significantly higher perioperative mortality risk.

Question

4. Which statements regarding elective treatment indications for aneurysms are correct?

a) The primary goal in treating an AAA is to prevent rupture.
b) The indication for treating an iliac aneurysm is to prevent peripheral embolization.
c) Aneurysms of visceral arteries are also treated to prevent rupture.
d) Aneurysms of visceral arteries are treated from a diameter of 2 cm.
e) Aneurysms of the popliteal artery (PopA) are also treated from a diameter of 2 cm to prevent rupture.

Answers

a) **Correct.** In AAA, the primary goal is to prevent rupture. The risk of rupture increases with diameter and is about 3% per year from 5.5 cm (from 5 cm in women). The growth rate is also important, so if the diameter increases by > 5 mm in 6 months, surgical intervention is also recommended.

b) **Incorrect.** For iliac aneurysms, the primary goal is also to prevent rupture. The current indication is a diameter of 3.5 cm or more. Previously, the threshold was 3 cm, but it was raised to 3.5 cm due to reduced rupture rates with improved BMT. In some cases, a size progression of > 3 mm in 6 months is defined as an indication for treatment, but this has not become common in clinical practice.

c) **Correct.** For visceral artery aneurysms (VAA), the primary indication for treatment is also to prevent rupture. Rupture of a VAA is life-threatening and has a very high mortality rate of up to 80%. However, the rupture rate of VAAs varies depending on location, being highest in aneurysms of the hepatic artery.
d) **Incorrect.** In principle, asymptomatic VAAs are treated from a diameter of 2 cm, as the annual risk of rupture rises to about 20%. However, there are exceptions. The most important exception is women of childbearing age: here, the indication for surgery is made upon diagnosis, regardless of absolute diameter. The reason is that pregnancy increases the risk of rupture, with high mortality for both mother and unborn child. False aneurysms are also treated invasively regardless of diameter, as their risk of rupture cannot be calculated.
e) **Incorrect.** The popliteal artery is treated from a diameter of 2 cm to prevent peripheral embolization or acute occlusion. Both result in acute ischemia and can lead to limb loss. The risk of amputation with acute popliteal artery occlusion is up to 50%. Rupture is extremely rare and, due to tamponade after bleeding into soft tissue, is not (or only in exceptional cases) life-threatening. If a popliteal aneurysm has no mural thrombus and the patient has a high surgical risk, the indication for invasive exclusion can be made only from 3 cm. Otherwise, a more liberal indication is recommended if there is a mural thrombus and already (usually asymptomatic) embolization into one or more lower leg vessels. Further diagnostics often reveal segmental or complete occlusion of lower leg vessels. If only one patent crural vessel remains with mural thrombus in the aneurysm, surgery is recommended from 1.5 cm.

Question

5. Which statements regarding abdominal aortic aneurysm (AAA) are correct?

a) In clinical practice, an aortic aneurysm is defined as a diameter of 3 cm or more.
b) The greatest risk factor for developing an aortic aneurysm is arterial hypertension.
c) The prevalence of abdominal aortic aneurysm in the population over 65 years is 10–15%.
d) Genetic diseases that can cause an aneurysm include Marfan, Ehlers-Danlos, and Loeys-Dietz syndromes.

e) Clinically, Loeys-Dietz syndrome manifests not only with aneurysm formation but also with skeletal, cardiovascular, and facial abnormalities. Typical distinguishing external features compared to Marfan syndrome are hypertelorism (abnormally wide distance between the eyes) and bifid uvula (split uvula at the end of the soft palate).

Answers

a) **Correct.** Between 2–3 cm is called ectasia, from 3 cm an aneurysm. Strictly speaking, the diameter of the proximal and distal normal-caliber aorta should be multiplied by 1.5 to define the threshold between ectasia and aneurysm. For simplicity, an aneurysm is defined as ≥ 3 cm, although for a tall, robust man (2.3 cm normal aorta) this would only apply from 3.5 cm, and for a small, thin woman (1.7 cm normal aorta) from 2.5 cm.
b) **Incorrect.** Nicotine abuse is the greatest risk factor for the development of AAA. The reasons are the progression of atherosclerotic plaque formation due to nicotine abuse. There is also increasing evidence that nicotine leads to increased expression and action of cytokines, resulting in an inflammatory process in the aortic vessel wall.
c) **Incorrect.** Prevalence increases with age and is 4% (women) to 7.7% (men) in the population aged 65 and older, with an average of 5.5%. The most common underlying disease is atherosclerosis; genetic diseases (connective tissue disorders), autoimmune diseases (inflammatory aneurysm), or infections (mycotic aneurysm) are much less common.
d) **Correct.** All three syndromes can clinically manifest with aortic aneurysms. In contrast to atherosclerotic aneurysms, these aneurysms occur at a younger age, often in the third or fourth decade of life.
e) **Correct.** Loeys-Dietz syndrome is often associated with chest deformities, foot malpositions, hyperextensible joints, and spinal curvature. Distinctive facial features include a cleft palate and ocular hypertelorism (abnormally wide distance between the eyes).

Question

6. Which statements regarding sonographic diagnosis and follow-up of AAA are correct?

a) Ultrasound is the most important diagnostic method for screening and follow-up.

b) There are no special requirements for the measurement method during follow-up.
c) The variability of diameter measurement in CT angiography varies little between different observers (inter-observer).
d) An 80-year-old patient with a 7 cm AAA who refuses surgery should be closely monitored with ultrasound every 3 months.
e) A patient with a 4 cm AAA should be monitored annually by ultrasound.

Answers

a) **Correct.** Abdominal ultrasound is one of the most important screening examinations and should be performed during general practitioner check-ups. This can significantly reduce AAA-associated mortality. The recommendation is a one-time ultrasound from age 65, and regardless of age in patients with a family history. If the aortic diameter is < 3 cm and there is no family history, further follow-up is not necessary.
b) **Incorrect.** Sonographic diameter measurements should always be performed in a standardized manner to avoid examiner-dependent measurement deviations. According to guideline recommendations, measurements should be taken strictly perpendicular from outer wall to outer wall (OTO, outer to outer). Other strictly perpendicular options are inner to inner (ITI) or leading edge to leading edge (LELE). The latter means ventral front (outer wall) to dorsal front (inner wall). Oblique diameter measurements should be strictly avoided, as they can lead to significant inaccuracies, especially in follow-up, resulting in misjudgment of size progression.
c) **Incorrect.** Diameter measurement using CT should also be standardized, as differences of 2–5 mm (or more) can occur between different observers. This can be significantly reduced by three-dimensional measurement methods.
d) **Incorrect.** If a patient refuses invasive treatment (either surgical or endovascular) of an AAA > 5.5 cm, this should be documented and communicated to relatives. Sonographic follow-up is unnecessary, as it would have no consequences. The patient's wishes should also be respected in the event of rupture, and emergency admission to the nearest hospital should be avoided.
e) **Correct.** The ESVS guideline recommends the following ultrasound follow-up intervals:
   I. 3–3.9 cm: every 3 years
   II. 4–4.9 cm: annually
   III. from 5 cm: every 3 to 6 months

Question

7. Which statements regarding iliac aneurysms are correct?

a) About 20% of patients with an AAA also have an iliac aneurysm.
b) The prevalence of iliac aneurysms is < 1%.
c) Typical symptoms of iliac aneurysms are abdominal pain and urinary retention.
d) Iliac aneurysms are classified according to Reber.
e) The in-hospital mortality of ruptured iliac aneurysm is higher than that of rAAA.

Answers

a) **False.** Involvement of the iliac arteries occurs in about 30–50%. This is also evident in the Allenberg classification. Here, in types IIB (15%) and IIC (30–35%), the iliac arteries are also affected. However, iliac aneurysms can also occur in isolation.
b) **Correct.** Isolated iliac aneurysms are very rare and occur with a prevalence of less than 1%. The most commonly affected vessel is the common iliac artery (AIC) (70%), much less frequently the internal iliac artery (AII) at 20%, and the external iliac artery (AIE) at 10%.
c) **Correct.** Typical symptoms include abdominal pain, lumbosacral nerve irritation, as well as urogenital problems such as bladder emptying disorders, hematuria, and infections of the kidneys and urinary tract. However, the majority of iliac aneurysms only become symptomatic at the stage of rupture and are therefore diagnosed late.
d) **Correct.** The basis of the Reber classification is the involvement of the individual segments AIC, AIE, and AII alone or in combination. Type I affects only the AIC, type II the isolated AII, type III AIC and AII, and in type IV all three segments are involved.
e) **Correct.** The mortality rate of ruptured iliac aneurysm is 70–100%, higher than that of rAAA, which is 40–80%. This may be due to the often more difficult and demanding management, especially of internal iliac aneurysms. Furthermore, ruptured iliac aneurysms usually have a larger diameter than rAAA, which can also lead to technical challenges. In addition, patients with iliac aneurysms are on average older than those with rAAA, which further explains the increased perioperative risk.

Question

8. Which statements about aortobiiliac endovascular treatment of infrarenal aortic aneurysms are correct?

a) Assessment of the access routes is part of the preoperative planning for endovascular aortic repair (EVAR) of infrarenal aortic aneurysms.
b) The iliac diameter (distal landing zone) is not relevant for the selection of the endoprosthesis.
c) The diameter in the aortic neck region (proximal landing zone) should not exceed 30 mm.
d) The length of the proximal landing zone should be at least 15 mm in uncomplicated EVAR.
e) The diameter and length of the iliac extensions should be determined preoperatively.

Answers

a) **Correct.** In endovascular procedures, assessment of the access routes is fundamentally extremely important to avoid intraoperative "surprises." For example, stenoses of the pelvic arteries may be overlooked, making passage with prosthetic materials impossible. This may necessitate aborting the surgical procedure or lead to serious complications, such as dissection or even rupture of the iliac arteries. The minimum diameter of the iliac arteries should not be less than 8 mm.
b) **False.** Not only the proximal but also the distal landing zone must meet certain morphological requirements. The diameter of the landing zone should not be > 25 mm and not shorter than 2 cm. Otherwise, the risk of developing a leak (type Ib endoleak) is very high. Common aortobiiliac endoprostheses have extensions (limbs) with a maximum diameter of up to 28 mm (e.g., Endurant II/IIs® from Medtronic).
c) **Correct.** The proximal diameter of common EVAR prostheses (e.g., Endurant II/IIs™ from Medtronic) ranges from 23 to 36 mm. Consequently, aneurysms with a neck diameter of up to 30 mm can be treated endovascularly without additional proximal fixation measures (e.g., Heli-FX™ EndoAnchor™ system).
d) **Correct.** The "neck length" in the proximal landing zone should not be less than 15 mm to allow anchoring of the prosthesis. In addition, the instructions for use (IFUs) of many manufacturers state that the neck should be

straight (not conical, straight with an angulation of < 60°) and free of calcifications and thrombotic deposits.

e) **Correct.** The diameter and length of the iliac extensions (limbs) should be measured and determined in advance. A selection of different prostheses should be available for the procedure.

a. Common lengths are 80–200 mm (e.g., Endurant II/IIs™ 82, 93, 124, 156, 199).
b. Common distal diameters range from 10 to 28 mm (e.g., Endurant II/IIs™: 10, 13, 16, 20, 24, 28 mm). The proximal diameter at the limbs is 16 mm, so that they anchor in the main body limb (14 mm).
c. Iliac extensions are available in
   i. straight (i.e., same diameter proximally and distally)
   ii. tapered (distally narrower than proximally)
   iii. flared (distally wider than proximally).

Question

9. Which statements about infrarenal aortic aneurysm are correct?

a) Abdominal aortic aneurysm (AAA) is located infrarenally in 80% of cases.
b) The infrarenal aorta in a 25-year-old man is physiologically larger in diameter than in a 65-year-old.
c) Smoking is the most important risk factor for the development of an aortic aneurysm.
d) In clinical practice, infrarenal aortic aneurysm is often classified according to Allenberg.
e) The greatest risk factor for rupture of a 6 cm aortic aneurysm is sex.

Answers

a) **False.** AAA is located infrarenally in 95% of cases; only 5% are above the renal arteries (suprarenal). According to data from the Aortic Registry of the German Institute for Vascular Medicine Health Research (DIGG), about 10% of infrarenal AAAs are classified as juxtarenal, which results in approximately 85% infrarenal, 10% juxtarenal, and 5% suprarenal. However, it should be noted that the definition is not applied uniformly. Officially, juxtarenal is defined as follows:

I. in **open repair**, at least temporarily, the aortic clamp is placed above one of the renal arteries, and

II. in **endovascular repair**, the aneurysm extends up to just below the renal arteries, but at least one scallop, fenestration, branch, or chimney/snorkel to a renal or visceral artery is required.

Regardless of the definition, it can be remembered that at least 85% of all abdominal aortic aneurysms are infrarenal and that neither open nor endovascular repair requires treatment of the renal arteries.

b) **False.** Physiologically, the infrarenal aorta in a 25-year-old man has a diameter of about 18 mm, which increases to up to 25 mm in a 65-year-old. An aneurysm is defined as a diameter of 30 mm or more. The physiological increase in diameter can be explained by the loss of elasticity that typically occurs with increasing age.

c) **Correct.** Smoking is the most decisive risk factor for the development of an aortic aneurysm, ranking ahead of arterial hypertension and diabetes mellitus. Patients with chronic obstructive pulmonary disease (COPD) also suffer more frequently from aortic aneurysms than those with healthy lungs, due to both nicotine abuse and often years of glucocorticoid use. The exact pathomechanism of aortic wall damage by nicotine is not fully understood, but there is significant evidence for nicotine-induced inhibition of collagen and elastin synthesis, resulting in decreased resistance and elasticity of the aortic wall. This is also considered an explanation for the significantly increased rupture rate in smokers.

d) **Correct.** The classification of infrarenal AAA according to Allenberg is widely used in clinical practice and is included in many operative reports. It is divided into types I–III, with only type III having a proximal distance < 1.5 cm to the renal arteries; in types I and II, the distance is > 1.5 cm. In type I, the distance to the aortic bifurcation is > 1 cm; in type II, a distinction is made between IIA: extends to the aortic bifurcation, IIB: extends to the middle of the common iliac artery, IIC: extends to the iliac bifurcation. In the original version of the classification, types IIC and III were considered indications for surgery, but this has changed with the increase in endovascular options.

e) **Correct.** The greatest independent risk factor for rupture of an AAA, in addition to maximum diameter, is sex: women have a fourfold higher risk of suffering a rupture than men. In addition, nicotine abuse doubles the risk of rupture. Patient age had no significant influence on rupture rate. However, this currently does not (yet) have consequences for the indication for invasive treatment; the development of the next guideline recommendations remains to be seen. Especially in women, the above-mentioned circumstance of a higher rupture rate may lead to a more generous and earlier indication for invasive aneurysm exclusion. Whether this will also lead to a change in the surgical indication for smokers is questionable. It must be considered that the majority of AAA patients are or were smokers and also have a higher perioperative complication risk (especially due to pulmonary and cardiac complications).

Question

10. Which statements about thoracic aortic aneurysm are correct?

a) Thoracic aortic aneurysm (TAA) is more common than abdominal aortic aneurysm (AAA).
b) Thoracic aortic aneurysm (TAA) affects men more often than women.
c) Thoracic aortic aneurysms (TAA) are only operated on at a diameter > 6 cm due to an increased perioperative complication rate.
d) TEVAR can be complicated by an aberrant right subclavian artery (A. lusoria).
e) Hoarseness can be the first sign of a thoracic aortic aneurysm (TAA).

Answers

a) **False.** TAA is much less common than AAA. The annual incidence of TAA is currently about 6 per 100,000, while that of AAA is 40 per 100,000.
b) **False.** Compared to AAA, TAA occurs more frequently in women than in men. In addition, affected women are on average 10–15 years older than men. Interestingly, women have a higher rupture rate, and more than one in three patients with a ruptured TAA is female.[1]
c) **False.** In arteriosclerotic TAA, the indication for invasive therapy is made at a diameter of 5.5 cm. This corresponds to the current standard surgical indication for AAA. In TAA caused by connective tissue disorders, including
   I. Marfan syndrome
   II. Ehlers-Danlos syndrome
   III. Loeys-Dietz syndrome

[1] Clouse WD, Hallett JW Jr, Schaff HV, Gayari MM, Ilstrup DM, Melton LJ 3rd. Improved prognosis of thoracic aortic aneurysms: a population-based study. JAMA. 1998 Dec 9;280(22):1926-9. https://doi.org/10.1001/jama.280.22.1926. PMID: 9851478.

the surgical indication is often made at 4.5 cm due to the increased risk of rupture. However, it must be considered that younger patients with connective tissue disorders have a lower perioperative mortality risk, as they do not have cardiovascular risk factors. However, TAAs in connective tissue disorders should initially be treated with open repair, and endovascular revision should only be considered in case of complications. Primary endovascular treatment should be avoided, as the long-term results of TEVAR are unsatisfactory in this special patient group due to often progressive and unpredictable aneurysm growth.

d) **Correct.** An aberrant origin of the right subclavian artery from the descending aorta (A. lusoria) can complicate endovascular treatment of a TAA. A. lusoria as a normal variant occurs in about 1% of cases; an aneurysmal dilation is referred to as a Kommerell diverticulum.
e) **Correct.** The most well-known clinical sign of a TAA is paravertebral pain. However, hoarseness can also be an initial clinical sign of a TAA if the recurrent laryngeal nerve (especially the left) is involved and compressed. Stridor due to tracheal compression, dyspnea due to lung compression, dysphagia due to esophageal compression, and superior vena cava syndrome due to compression of the superior vena cava can also be clinical signs of a TAA.

Question

11. Which statements about popliteal aneurysm are correct?

a) About one in five patients with an AAA also has an aneurysm of the popliteal artery.
b) More than half of patients with bilateral popliteal artery aneurysms have an AAA.
c) Aneurysm of the popliteal artery affects almost exclusively men.
d) Every second patient with an acutely thrombosed popliteal artery aneurysm will eventually require above-knee amputation.
e) Popliteal aneurysm should be treated electively at an early stage to prevent rupture.

Answers

a) **Correct.** About 20% of patients with an AAA also have a popliteal artery aneurysm. For this reason, it is recommended that every patient with an aortic aneurysm also undergo an ultrasound of the popliteal fossa to rule out or avoid missing a popliteal artery aneurysm.

b) **Correct.** About 70% of patients with bilateral popliteal artery aneurysms also have an aortic aneurysm. Therefore, when a popliteal aneurysm is diagnosed, an ultrasound of the aorta or a CTA of the entire aorta should be performed.
c) **Correct.** Popliteal aneurysm is the most common peripheral aneurysm, but still a very rare disease with an estimated prevalence of 1% in men over 65 years of age. Women are extremely rarely affected; literature reports on popliteal aneurysm are, with few exceptions, about men. The reasons for this are unknown.
d) **Correct.** The risk of limb loss in acutely occluded popliteal aneurysm is up to 50%. Especially in cases with prior embolization into the lower leg arteries and poor outflow, the chances of successful bypass reconstruction are low. Although popliteal aneurysm is rarely life-threatening compared to aortic aneurysm, it is still a very serious condition. Therefore, elective therapy should be considered at a maximum diameter of 2 cm at the latest. If only one native outflow vessel remains in the lower leg, a more generous indication is recommended at a diameter of 1.5 cm.
e) **False.** The main risk of a popliteal aneurysm is peripheral embolization and acute thrombotic occlusion. Peripheral embolization is often asymptomatic, as collateralization through unaffected lower leg vessels is usually sufficient. Only when this is no longer adequate, the third crural vessel is affected, or the aneurysm is completely thrombosed, do patients become symptomatic. Therefore, in popliteal aneurysm, the aim is to prevent peripheral embolization, not the extremely rare rupture. Most popliteal aneurysms present with chronic or acute circulatory disturbance.

Question

12. Which statements about venous aneurysms are correct?

a) Venous aneurysms are a very rare disease.
b) The most feared complication is rupture.
c) The most common location is the popliteal vein.
d) Patients usually become symptomatic due to swelling in the popliteal fossa.
e) Conservative therapy is the treatment of choice for venous popliteal aneurysm.

Answers

a) **Correct.** Venous aneurysms have an estimated prevalence of less than 0.1%; most scientific reports are case reports or small case series.
b) **False.** Venous aneurysms very rarely rupture.

c) **Correct.** Most of the rare case reports in the literature concern aneurysm of the popliteal vein.
d) **False.** Most patients become symptomatic due to thrombosis with or without pulmonary embolism.
e) **False.** Due to the risk of thrombosis with pulmonary embolism, surgical aneurysmorrhaphy, interposition, or patch plasty should be indicated upon diagnosis. Only small aneurysms and accompanying multimorbidity with high perioperative risk justify conservative follow-up.

Question

13. Which statements about the prevalence of aortic aneurysms are correct?

a) About 3–5% of men over 65 years of age in Germany have an AAA.
b) AAA is much more common than thoracic aortic aneurysm (TAA).
c) Women do not need "aortic screening" because aneurysms are rare in this group.
d) Connective tissue disorders account for about 20% of AAA.
e) About 20% of patients with an AAA also have a thoracic AA.

Answers

a) **Correct.** The prevalence of AAA in men over 65 years of age is about 3–5%; the male-to-female ratio is about 6:1. Women are much less frequently affected, and the reasons for this are unclear. Hormonal protection by estrogens is suspected.
b) **Correct.** TAA has a prevalence of 0.3–0.5% in the general population and is therefore much less common than AAA. In other words, AAA is a relatively rare disease, but about 10 times more common than TAA. In patients with connective tissue disorders (Marfan, Ehlers-Danlos, and Loeys-Dietz syndromes), the situation is different: these patients develop TAA more frequently, especially in the ascending aorta and aortic arch. In addition, the risk of rupture in this patient group is significantly higher than in atherosclerotic aneurysms.
c) **False.** Women are six times less likely to have an AAA than men, but have a fourfold higher risk of rupture. Therefore, the guidelines of the German Society for Vascular Surgery now recommend aortic screening from age 65 for women with risk factors
   I. Current or former smoker,
   II. High blood pressure,
   III. Vascular disease in first-degree relatives with vascular aneurysm

from age 65.

d) **False.** More than 90% of AAAs are due to atherosclerosis; the remaining 10% are caused by inflammation (mycotic aneurysms) and connective tissue disorders (Marfan, Ehlers-Danlos, and Loeys-Dietz syndromes). Aortic dissection can also lead to wall weakness and thus a dissecting aneurysm, but even in these cases, atherosclerosis is mostly the underlying cause of the dissection.

e) **False.** In about 10% of cases, patients diagnosed with AAA also have a thoracic aneurysm. Therefore, especially at the initial diagnosis of AAA, it is recommended to image the entire aorta by CTA to avoid missing or to rule out thoracic aneurysms.

Question

14. Which statements about the rupture rate of an AAA are correct?

a) The rupture rate of an AAA is higher in smokers than in non-smokers.

b) An asymptomatic AAA with a diameter > 8 cm has an annual rupture risk of 10%.

c) Ruptured AAAs often present to the emergency department in the early morning hours.

d) The use of steroids and immunosuppressants increases the rupture risk of AAA.

e) Metformin can reduce the rupture risk of an AAA.

Answers

a) **Correct.** Nicotine abuse significantly increases the rupture risk of an AAA, which is attributed to reduced wall stability and rapid increase in size. Other independent risk factors include female sex, arterial hypertension, and a diameter > 6 cm. In addition, patients with connective tissue disorders also have an increased rupture risk, which is why the indication for surgical intervention is made individually and earlier in these cases.

b) **Incorrect.** An AAA with a diameter > 8 cm has an annual rupture risk of > 60%. The rupture risk increases exponentially with diameter and is

I. 4–5 cm: 1–5%
II. 5–6 cm: 10%
III. 6–7 cm: 20%
IV. 7–8 cm: 40%
V. >8 cm: > 60%.

c) **Correct.** Rupture of an AAA often occurs in the context of blood pressure spikes, which typically happen at night when getting up to use the bathroom. Of course, hypertensive crises can also occur during the day in stressful situations, especially in working patients. Pausing antihypertensive medications (intentionally or accidentally) can also lead to hypertensive crises and an increased rupture rate.
d) **Correct.** The use of steroids and immunosuppressants clearly weakens the aortic wall, which is explained by impaired synthesis of stable connective tissue. Consequently, patients on chronic steroid medication (e.g., asthma patients) should be treated invasively more liberally and, if justifiable, at an earlier stage. In addition, coughing fits can lead to increased abdominal pressure or pressure spikes, which may further increase the rupture risk.
e) **Incorrect.** Although metformin appears to have an inhibitory effect on the development and growth of abdominal aortic aneurysms, it does not reduce the rupture risk. This protective effect of metformin is currently being investigated in two European multicenter RCTs:
   I. in the Swedish MAAAGI study (Metformin for Abdominal Aortic Aneurysm Growth Inhibition) (open randomized controlled trial) and
   II. in the Vienna-MetAAA study initiated in Austria

   Risk factors for rupture, in addition to the absolute diameter (which is often the main factor and decisive for invasive therapy), include, among others:
   1. rapid increase in aortic diameter by more than 1 cm per year (or > 5 mm/6 months)
   2. hemorrhage into the thrombus
   3. disrupted calcified rings in the aneurysm wall
   4. saccular outpouchings of the aortic wall
   5. connective tissue disorders (Marfan syndrome, Ehlers-Danlos syndrome, Loeys-Dietz syndrome)
   6. female sex
   7. use of steroids and immunosuppressants
   8. poorly controlled arterial hypertension

Question

15. Which statements about the surgical indication for abdominal aortic aneurysm (AAA) are correct?

a) A surgical indication exists for men with an absolute diameter of 5 cm.
b) Regardless of the maximum diameter of an AAA, a surgical indication exists if there is a size progression of 10 mm in 6 months.

c) Every symptomatic aneurysm should be treated invasively.
d) The rupture risk of an AAA exceeds the perioperative mortality/lethality risk from 5.5 cm onwards.
e) Even a hemodynamically unstable patient with a malignant underlying disease should at least receive endovascular treatment for a ruptured AAA.

Answers

a) **Incorrect.** Previously, 5 cm was considered the "magic" threshold. Nowadays, the indication for invasive therapy is made later, namely only from a maximum diameter of 5.5 cm (from 5 cm in small, slender women). The reason for this is the better outcomes with conservative therapy using BMT. This has led to a reduction in rupture risk in recent years.
b) **Incorrect.** A surgical indication exists for a size progression of 5 mm/6 months or 10 mm in 1 year. This applies regardless of the absolute diameter, which is why regular monitoring is important. It is also important that diameters are measured in a standardized way, ideally by the same examiner. Otherwise, measurement inaccuracies can lead to serious misjudgments.
c) **Correct.** Pain attributable to the aneurysm (typically pressure pain over the pulsation and back pain) must always prompt exclusion, otherwise the rupture risk is very high. Ultimately, even a 3 cm aneurysm should be excluded if it causes pain and is thus symptomatic. In clinical practice, however, this is very rare; pain is typically caused by a correspondingly large aneurysm. Nevertheless, "small" aneurysms with typical pain symptoms should be taken seriously and, until proven otherwise, considered "symptomatic" and treated accordingly.
d) **Correct**. The rupture risk for aneurysms < 5 cm is about 1–3% and then increases exponentially. The annual rupture rate, depending on size, is
   I. 6 cm: about 10%
   II. 7 cm: about 20%
   III. 8 cm: about 40%
e) **Incorrect.** When determining the indication for surgery, the patient's wishes, underlying diseases, and estimated remaining life expectancy must also be considered. There are also not infrequently patients who, despite a known aneurysm and an elective surgical indication, have refused an invasive procedure. This previously expressed wish must also be respected in the event of rupture if the patient is no longer able to communicate. Therefore, environmental diagnostics and discussions with relatives should always be sought in advance. In a hemodynamically unstable, possibly

already intubated patient with a malignant underlying disease (e.g., colon carcinoma), extreme caution should be exercised regarding surgical intervention for both medical and ethical reasons.

Question

16. Which statements about the surgical indication and choice of procedure for popliteal aneurysm (PopA) are correct?

a) For asymptomatic popliteal aneurysms (PopA), a surgical indication generally exists from 2.0 cm.
b) For a popliteal aneurysm (PopA) with good morphology, endovascular treatment should primarily be recommended.
c) In acutely occluded popliteal aneurysms (PopA) with Rutherford IIB limb ischemia and good morphology, aspiration thrombectomy and stent implantation are recommended.
d) "Good morphology" in popliteal aneurysm (PopA) is defined as landing zones > 3 cm.
e) The lateral and posterior approaches for popliteal aneurysm (PopA) are equivalent.

Answers

a) **Incorrect.** The surgical indication for asymptomatic PopA is usually made at a maximum diameter of 2 cm, but in special cases it can be made as early as 1.5 cm or as late as 3 cm.
   I. **from 2.0 cm:**
      a) asymptomatic
      b) >1 patent lower leg artery
   II. **from 1.5 cm:**
      a) if the aneurysm contains a mural thrombus and
      b) has already (possibly silently) embolized into the lower leg arteries and
      c) only one lower leg artery remains perfused
   III. **from 3 cm:**
      a) without thrombus
      b) high perioperative risk
      c) reoperation

b) **Incorrect.** For a PopA with an indication for invasive therapy and suitable morphology, both endovascular and open approaches can be performed.
   I. Arguments for the open approach include
      a) good anesthesia tolerance and resilience
      b) remaining life expectancy > 5 years
      c) suitable GSV
   II. Arguments for the endovascular approach include
      a) combination with intra-arterial thrombolysis
      b) estimated life expectancy < 5 years
      c) multimorbidity
      d) reoperation
      e) no suitable vein material

   Primary patency rates (i.e., patency without the need for corrective interventions) are better with the open approach than with the endovascular approach; for secondary patency, there are no longer significant differences.
c) **Incorrect.** In the case of acute occlusion of a PopA, immediate surgical reconstruction should be performed to minimize the time to reperfusion. In addition, fasciotomy should always be performed, as this is necessary in the majority of patients due to poor or absent collateralization. The risk of limb loss is very high in acutely thrombosed PopA and ranges from 30–80%.
d) **Incorrect.** For PopA, the proximal and distal landing zones should each be > 15 mm long and free of aneurysm. It is also advisable to assess outflow to be prepared for any necessary peripheral interventions.
e) **Incorrect.** For short aneurysms in the P2 segment of the popliteal artery, the posterior approach should be preferred according to guidelines. However, if the aneurysm extends to the adductor canal, the lateral approach is recommended, as this facilitates proximal dissection.

Question

17. Which statements about endovascular aortic repair are correct?

a) The "chimney technique" of endovascular aortic repair is a further development of the "branched" technique.
b) With the "chimney technique" (Ch-EVAR), a type Ia endoleak occurs in > 25% of cases.
c) In endovascular repair of a suprarenal AAA, branched prostheses (bEVAR) are often used.

d) Type Ic endoleak describes a leak in fEVAR or bEVAR.
e) Long-segment thoracic endovascular aortic repair (TEVAR) carries a paraplegia risk of 20%.

Answers

a) **Incorrect.** The chimney technique, first described in 2003, is a “bailout” procedure for para- or suprarenal abdominal aortic aneurysms (AAA) or infrarenal AAAs with a short neck. The principle of the chimney technique (chimney = snorkel) is the insertion of covered stents (e.g., ViaBahn® by WL Gore) into the renal and, if necessary, visceral arteries from the subclavian approach, followed by standard EVAR implantation from the femoral approach. The chimneys then lie like snorkels alongside the main body and maintain renovisceral perfusion. The common abbreviation for this procedure is Ch-EVAR. It is an alternative to so-called branched prostheses, in which the stents do not lie alongside the main body but are passed through openings (fenestrations) and placed in the target vessel. However, as mentioned, it is considered a “bailout” procedure for difficult anatomy, not a further development of branched prostheses. In the case of type Ia endoleak after EVAR, the chimney technique is a possible treatment option and has already been used successfully.
b) **Incorrect.** The risk of a type Ia endoleak after Ch-EVAR is less than 10%. This is shown by data from the PERICLES registry study.[2] A distinction is also made between high-flow (HF) and low-flow (LF) type Ia endoleaks. In HF, contrast medium leaks immediately after application and fills the aneurysm sac antegradely; in LF, it occurs much later, in the late phase after contrast application. LF endoleaks usually seal themselves after a short time and are thus of little clinical relevance, as they can be managed conservatively. HF endoleaks, on the other hand, always require immediate invasive revision.

[2] Donas KP, Lee JT, Lachat M, Torsello G, Veith FJ; PERICLES investigators. Collected world experience about the performance of the snorkel/chimney endovascular technique in the treatment of complex aortic pathologies: the PERICLES registry. Ann Surg. 2015 Sep;262(3):546–53; discussion 552–3. https://doi.org/10.1097/SLA.0000000000001405. PMID: 26258324.

c) **Incorrect.** For suprarenal AAA, fenestrated prostheses (fEVAR) are often used, whereas for thoracoabdominal aortic aneurysm (TAAA), branched prostheses (bEVAR) are preferred. The indication for both types of prostheses is an insufficient proximal anchoring or landing zone. In AAA, the neck is too short, so the anchoring zone of the prosthesis must be extended proximally. This is achieved by fenestrations in the prosthesis, through which stents are implanted into the target vessels. This allows the main body to be anchored proximally to the origin of the renovisceral vessels, and through the fenestrations, stents maintain perfusion of the vessels located in the anchoring area.
Branched prostheses (bEVAR), on the other hand, have "arms" or branches instead of fenestrations, through which, similar to the fenestrated approach, extension stents are implanted into the target vessels. Branches are always necessary when the target vessels originate from the aneurysm and are not located in the "neck area." This bridges the distance from the main body to the target vessel, thereby reducing the risk of endoleaks.
d) **Correct.** Endoleaks are classified as types I–IV, with type I further subdivided into Ia-c:
   I. Endoleak in the anchoring area of the prosthesis components
      a) proximal anchoring
      b) distal anchoring
      c) anchoring in the area of renovisceral stent extensions
   II. Retrograde flow from side branches (usually lumbar arteries)
   III. Leakage at the overlap of prosthesis components (iliac extension)
   IV. Porosity of the prosthesis

   Type Ic endoleak thus refers to a leak in the area of the extension of stents into the renovisceral vessels.
e) **Correct.** TEVAR for long-segment lesions (aneurysm, dissection) is now considered the therapy of choice due to significantly reduced perioperative morbidity and mortality. It is less invasive than open aortic replacement, which often requires thoracotomy and sternotomy as well as the use of a heart-lung machine. Nevertheless, the endovascular approach also carries specific risks, including paraplegia. This risk increases with the length of the treated aortic segment and is up to 20% for long-segment TEVAR. This should be considered when choosing the prosthesis. Overstenting of the Adamkiewicz artery (A. radicularis magna) should be avoided, as it is the main artery supplying the spinal cord. However, its origin from the thoracic aorta is highly variable and preoperative visualization is rarely possible.

Question

18. Which statements about Marfan syndrome are correct?

a) An AAA in Marfan patients should preferably be treated endovascularly.
b) β-blockers are contraindicated in patients with Marfan syndrome and aortic aneurysms.
c) Statins are not indicated in Marfan patients with aortic aneurysm.
d) Marfan syndrome is the most common of the three connective tissue disorders associated with aortic aneurysms.
e) The life expectancy of untreated Marfan patients is about 30 years.

Answers

a) **Incorrect.** Aneurysms in connective tissue disorders such as Marfan, Loeys-Dietz, and Ehlers-Danlos syndromes should, according to guidelines, be treated with open surgery as the first intervention. For reoperations, the endovascular approach is preferred. According to current knowledge, the long-term results of open surgery are superior to the endovascular approach, which is why younger patients in particular benefit from open aortic replacement. Since patients with aneurysms requiring treatment due to congenital connective tissue disorders are usually much younger than aneurysm patients with atherosclerosis, the procedure with better and more reliable long-term results is preferred.
b) **Incorrect.** On the contrary, Marfan patients should receive β-blocker therapy to reduce the pressure load on the aorta. This is achieved through the negative inotropic, dromotropic, and chronotropic effects of β-blockers.
c) **Incorrect.** Even in patients with connective tissue disorders, administration of statins (pravastatin) has been shown to significantly slow the growth of aortic aneurysms. The exact mechanism, however, is unclear.
d) **Correct.** The three best-known, but still individually very rare, connective tissue disorders associated with aortic aneurysms are Marfan, Ehlers-Danlos, and Loeys-Dietz syndromes. The prevalence of Marfan syndrome is about 1:10,000, while Loeys-Dietz and Ehlers-Danlos syndromes have a prevalence of 1:100,000 to 1:1,000,000. Nevertheless, genetically determined aortopathies should not be underestimated.
e) **Correct.** Without therapy, the average life expectancy of Marfan patients is only 30 years. The most common causes of death are cardiovascular diseases, especially aortic pathologies and fatal ruptures. With early therapy

using antihypertensive medication (β-blockers, AT-I antagonists, or ACE inhibitors) and surgical exclusion of aortic (usually thoracic) aneurysms, life expectancy exceeds 60 years.

Question

19. Which statements about Ehlers-Danlos syndrome (EDS) are correct?

a) The characteristic feature of Ehlers-Danlos syndrome (EDS) is hyperextensibility of the skin.
b) Ehlers-Danlos syndrome (EDS) is divided into several subtypes, including a vascular type.
c) The life expectancy of patients with Ehlers-Danlos syndrome (EDS) of the vascular type is not reduced if aortic aneurysms are excluded at an early stage.
d) In young patients with dissection or rupture of peripheral arteries after minor trauma, e.g., iliac or femoral, EDS may be the underlying cause.
e) The guidelines of the ESC and ESVS provide clear recommendations for the indication to exclude aortic aneurysms in Ehlers-Danlos syndrome (EDS).

Answers

a) **Correct.** EDS typically presents with hyperextensible skin, which is due to a collagen synthesis disorder. This is the most striking feature of the disease, by which patients can often be recognized even without extensive additional investigations. Other features include hypermobility of joints, which is particularly noticeable and evident in the finger and toe joints.
b) **Correct.** EDS has several subtypes, including the classic type, a vascular type, hypermobile type, etc. The vascular type is inherited in an autosomal dominant manner and, in addition to the classic skin hyperextensibility, is associated with a pronounced tendency to hematomas and bleeding complications. In addition to the tendency to develop aortic aneurysms, these patients also have an above-average frequency of aneurysms in other vessels (e.g., visceral arteries) and suffer from varicosis.
c) **Incorrect.** Patients with EDS have a reduced life expectancy of about 50 years. Common causes of death, in addition to rupture of aortic aneurysms, include uterine rupture, rupture of visceral aneurysms, or rupture of intestinal structures. Surgical interventions in these patients are also associated

with an increased risk of complications, particularly bleeding. Therefore, while the indication for exclusion of any aneurysm should be made generously, the increased perioperative risk of complications must also be taken into account.

d) **Correct.** For a traumatic dissection or rupture of "healthy" vessels, a correspondingly severe trauma must usually have occurred and affected the arterial wall. This can be the case, for example, with comminuted fractures or massive joint dislocations. Dissections after minor trauma are suspicious for a pre-existing lesion and/or connective tissue disease, which should be ruled out.

e) **Incorrect.** There is no clear recommendation regarding the maximum diameter and growth rate of aortic aneurysms in EDS. Recommendations are often based on those for the management of aneurysms in Marfan syndrome. However, in elective treatment, the significantly increased perioperative bleeding risk in patients with vascular EDS (type IV) must be considered. In addition, surgical management of EDS patients with aortic aneurysms often falls within the field of cardiac surgery, as aneurysms of the ascending aorta and, less frequently, the descending aorta are most common. Thoracoabdominal aortic aneurysms are rare. Elective repair of an AAA in EDS patients should be considered at a maximum diameter of 5.5 cm (i.e., equivalent to an atherosclerotic aneurysm). There is a clear recommendation in the ESVS guidelines regarding conservative therapy, namely medical blood pressure control with β-blockers, but not for surgical indications.

Question

20. Which statements about Loeys-Dietz syndrome are correct?

a) Aortic dissections are a typical complication of Loeys-Dietz syndrome (LDS).
b) A distinctive feature of patients with Loeys-Dietz syndrome (LDS) is a bifid uvula.
c) Loeys-Dietz syndrome (LDS) has a prevalence of 1:100,000.
d) Aneurysms in Loeys-Dietz syndrome (LDS) preferentially occur in the abdominal aorta.
e) The indication for invasive exclusion of a thoracic aortic aneurysm in patients with Loeys-Dietz syndrome is given at 3 cm.

Answers

a) **Correct.** LDS typically involves disease of the thoracic, especially the proximal aorta. Dissections and aneurysms occur preferentially, and have even been described in children in individual cases. It is a potentially life-threatening disease that requires early cardiac and vascular surgical intervention.
b) **Correct.** Loeys-Dietz syndrome, along with Ehlers-Danlos and Marfan syndrome, is one of the congenital connective tissue disorders associated with an increased risk of developing aortic and peripheral aneurysms. The so-called uvula bifida is a characteristic of patients with Loeys-Dietz syndrome. This is a longitudinal split of the uvula, which is the mildest form of cleft lip and palate. Other clinical signs include craniofacial abnormalities, hypertelorism (increased distance between the eyes), and hypermobility of joints.
c) **Incorrect.** LDS has a prevalence of 1:1,000,000, with fewer than 100 case reports worldwide in the literature. The mode of inheritance, as with Marfan and Ehlers-Danlos syndrome, is autosomal dominant, which is common in connective tissue disorders.
d) **Incorrect.** In LDS, aortic disease (dissection and aneurysm) preferentially occurs in the thoracic segment, rarely in the abdominal or peripheral segments.
e) **Incorrect.** The surgical indication for exclusion of aortic aneurysms in patients with connective tissue disorders is made earlier than for atherosclerotic aneurysms, but not as early as 3 cm. Valve-sparing replacement of an ascending aortic aneurysm is recommended at a diameter of 4.5 cm, and replacement of the aortic arch or descending aorta at 4 cm.

Question

21. Which statements about ongoing studies on aortic aneurysms are correct?

a) The CAESAR study addresses the question of whether EVAR is better than conservative therapy for small aneurysms.
b) The ENCHANT study investigates the safety and success of TEVAR for aortic arch aneurysms.
c) The EXCeL study investigates the Excluder prosthesis from WL Gore in cases of challenging anatomy.

d) The LIMIT study investigates the limits of endovascular treatment of AAAs.
e) The ADVANCE study compares the stent grafts from WL Gore (Excluder®) and Medtronic (Endurant®).

Answers

a) **Correct.** The CAESAR study (Comparison of Surveillance Versus Aortic Endografting for small aneurysm repair) is a multicenter RCT in which small aneurysms with a diameter of 4.0–5.4 cm and a size progression of < 1 cm/year are either monitored by ultrasound or treated endovascularly. Twenty centers participated, and 360 patients were enrolled (182 vs. 178). After 4 years of follow-up, there was no significant difference in survival between the conservatively and operatively (endovascularly) treated groups, so the recommendation for endovascular treatment remains unchanged at a maximum diameter of 5.5 cm or a size progression of > 1 cm/year. The lower perioperative morbidity and mortality rates did not change this recommendation.
b) **Incorrect.** The ENCHANT study (**En**durant **CH**ev**A**r **N**ew Indication **T**rial) investigates the safety and success of endovascular treatment of juxtarenal abdominal aortic aneurysms (AAA) using the chimney technique. It is a multicenter study in Europe, the former Soviet Union, and the United Kingdom, with a planned enrollment of 150 patients. There is no control group, but the study aims to compare outcomes with branched or fenestrated prostheses. Advantages of the chimney technique include easier availability of these prostheses, as custom manufacturing is not required. However, the safety of this technique is criticized, as it always requires a supra-aortic access. The issue of type I endoleaks is also a focus of interest.
c) **Correct.** The EXCeL study is a multicenter study in Europe and the United Kingdom, aiming to investigate and document the applicability and outcomes of the GORE® EXCLUDER® Conformable AAA Endoprosthesis in more detail. The focus is particularly on use in challenging anatomy, meaning use at or beyond the limits of the IFUs (instructions for use). The configuration of the neck is of particular interest, with the following recommendations:
   I. Neck length > 10 mm with infrarenal angulation < 60°, and
   II. Neck length > 15 mm with infrarenal angulation < 90°.
d) **Incorrect.** The LIMIT study (LIMItIng AAA With meTformin) is a multicenter study investigating the effect of metformin medication on the growth of abdominal aortic aneurysms. Smaller studies have already provided

initial evidence that metformin inhibits the growth and size progression of AAA, although the exact mechanism is unclear. The LIMIT study was initiated to investigate this effect in a randomized design. The metformin dose is initially 500 mg/day, which is increased to 1000 mg twice daily if well tolerated, and compared with placebo. Nearly 500 patients are to be enrolled; inclusion criteria include age > 55, no diabetes or diabetes medication, and an aortic diameter > 35 mm and < 50 mm. Planned follow-up is initially 2 years; diameters are documented by CT scans.

e) **Correct.** The ADVANCE study is a randomized multicenter study comparing the applicability and success of the Endurant II/IIs® prosthesis with the Excluder® endoprosthesis for infrarenal AAA. Five hundred patients are to be enrolled, with a follow-up of 5 years. Hospitals in Europe, Japan, and the United States can participate; the study is sponsored by Medtronic.

Question

22. Which statements about major completed aneurysm studies are correct?

a) An important question in studies on aortic aneurysms is the comparison between open and endovascular repair.
b) The POPART study is an RCT comparing open versus endovascular repair of popliteal aneurysms.
c) The PiERO study compared percutaneous femoral access with open (cut down) access in EVAR.
d) There is a large multicenter RCT comparing open and endovascular repair of visceral artery aneurysms.
e) Due to the urgency of treatment, there has so far been no study comparing open and endovascular repair in rAAA.

Answers

a) **Correct.** Many studies on aortic aneurysms focus on the comparison between open and endovascular repair. Four frequently cited multicenter RCTs are:
   I. EVAR (endovascular versus open repair of abdominal aortic aneurysm)
   II. DREAM (Dutch Randomised Endovascular Aneurysm Management)
   III. OVER (Open Versus Endovascular Repair)
   IV. ACE (Anévrysme de l'aorte abdominale Chirurgie versus Endoprothèse)

The perioperative complication rate (30-day mortality) and follow-up results (reintervention rate) were compared. As expected, the 30-day mortality after open repair was higher (1–5%) than after endovascular repair (about 1%), whereas the reintervention rate was higher with endovascular repair (5–10%) than with open surgery (2–5%). Only in the ACE study was the 30-day mortality lower after open repair (1%) than after endovascular repair (1–2%).

b) **Incorrect.** The POPART study is a registry study on the treatment situation and outcomes of popliteal aneurysm repair in Germany. An RCT has not yet been conducted due to the rarity of the condition. In the POPART study, as expected, the hospital stay was significantly shorter after EVAR (5–7 days) than after open repair (OR) (10 days). The primary patency rates after 1 and 2 years were better after OR (85% and 45%) than after EVAR (75% and 30%). The primary patency rate after 12 months was also significantly better with vein interposition grafts (90%) than with synthetic grafts (70%).
c) **Correct.** The PiERO study (percutaneous versus open access in endovascular aneurysm repair) was a multicenter randomized trial comparing percutaneous and open femoral access in EVAR procedures. There was a significant reduction in postoperative pain after percutaneous access; however, there was no significant difference in wound healing or risk of wound infection.
d) **Incorrect.** Due to the rarity of visceral artery aneurysms, with a prevalence of about 0.1%, no RCT has been initiated or conducted to date. Several single-center clinical studies have investigated outcomes after treatment of visceral aneurysms, but with retrospective study designs. The research questions included outcomes after open and endovascular repair, particularly with regard to different techniques and materials.
e) **Incorrect.** There is a multicenter RCT comparing EVAR and OR in rAAA. This is the so-called IMPROVE study (Immediate Management Of Patients with Rupture: Open Versus Endovascular). In 29 centers (United Kingdom), more than 600 patients with rAAA were enrolled and, if suitable morphology was present, treated either by open surgery (n=297) or endovascularly (n=316). The 30-day mortality was about 40% for both procedures, and costs were also comparable. After endovascular therapy, significantly more patients (94%) could be discharged home than after open repair (70%). In addition, after 3 years of follow-up, the endovascularly treated patient group had a significantly better quality of life.

Hemodialysis Shunts

7

Question

1. Which statements regarding the NKF-KDOQI guidelines (National Kidney Foundation-Kidney Disease Outcomes Quality Initiative) are correct?

a) Before creating a Cimino shunt, excessive fluid removal during hemodialysis should be avoided.
b) No more than 10% of patients with end-stage renal disease should be permanently dialyzed via an atrial catheter.
c) According to the NKF-KDOQI recommendations, a non-tunneled CVC (Shaldon catheter) should be left in place for a maximum of 4 weeks.
d) According to NKF-KDOQI recommendations, patients with end-stage renal disease who will receive a living donor transplant within 90 days should still receive an autologous shunt.
e) According to NKF-KDOQI guideline recommendations, exchanging a CVC using the Seldinger technique should be avoided for infection prophylaxis.

Answers

a) **Correct.** Experience shows that overly aggressive fluid removal carries a high risk of perioperative hypotension, which can lead to acute thrombosis of the shunt vein at the newly created anastomosis. This can be the cause of immediate occlusion, especially in peripheral shunts (such as the Cimino shunt) with small-caliber vessels.

S. Regus, *Vascular Surgery: Questions and Answers*,
https://doi.org/10.1007/978-3-662-73387-5_7

b) **Correct.** According to current guideline recommendations, no more than 10% of hemodialysis patients should be permanently dialyzed with an atrial catheter. Currently, > 90% of patients with acute renal failure and approximately 60–80% of patients with chronic renal failure are initially dialyzed via a Demers catheter. Improved access planning and interdisciplinary collaboration between nephrologists and vascular surgeons should aim for a significant reduction in catheter placements. The greatest potential for reducing catheter placements lies in the timely creation of arteriovenous fistulas, so that the maturation phase occurs in the pre-terminal stage and catheter placement becomes unnecessary.

c) **Incorrect.** According to NKF-KDOQI recommendations (expert opinion), a non-tunneled CVC should be left in situ for a maximum of 2 weeks. Otherwise, the risk of infection increases significantly, further endangering patients who are often already immunosuppressed and multimorbid. Therefore, early conversion to a tunneled catheter is recommended. If the end of dialysis dependency is not foreseeable, the highest priority must also be given to the early creation of a dialysis shunt (ideally autologous).

d) **Incorrect.** The NKF-KDOQI guidelines indicate the use of an atrial catheter in this situation to bridge the waiting period until transplantation. Other indications for short-term catheter dialysis, according to expert opinion, include

   I. a dialysis shunt that has already been created but is not yet usable
      – maturation period not yet completed
      – significant soft tissue swelling
      – hematoma (postoperative or after unsuccessful puncture attempt)
      – infection (impending or manifest, especially with synthetic shunts)
   II. impending or acute rejection of a kidney transplant
   III. temporarily unusable peritoneal catheter

e) **Incorrect.** There is no clear evidence that exchanging an indwelling CVC using the Seldinger technique is associated with an increased risk of infection. This situation often arises when converting from a non-tunneled to a tunneled CVC. No increased infection risk has been observed after "over-the-wire" exchange. However, if there is redness at the catheter exit site or infection of the soft tissue, "over-the-wire" exchange should be avoided and the tunneled CVC should be implanted on the contralateral side. Ideally, the suspicious non-tunneled catheter should be removed before implantation of the new catheter, as far as this can be organized with the dialysis schedule.

Question

2. Which statements regarding atrial catheters are correct?

a) For acute dialysis, a Shaldon catheter is often placed via the subclavian vein (SV).
b) To bridge the maturation period of a hemodialysis shunt, the patient can be discharged from inpatient care with a functioning Shaldon catheter and continue as an outpatient.
c) The only difference between atrial catheters and central venous catheters is the diameter.
d) A functioning Demers catheter should remain in situ as long as possible, even with a well-functioning hemodialysis shunt, to ensure immediate access in case of shunt occlusion.
e) In Germany, initial dialysis for end-stage renal disease is performed in 50% of patients via an atrial catheter and in 50% via a native AV fistula.

Answers

a) **Incorrect.** A Shaldon catheter is used only for short-term hemodialysis, usually in the intensive care unit by intensivists. It is a large-bore polyurethane or silicone catheter, inserted percutaneously using the Seldinger technique and non-tunneled, preferably via the internal jugular vein (IJV). The tip is positioned in front of the right atrium, which is checked radiologically. The right IJV is preferred over the left if it has sufficient lumen and is patent, due to the shorter distance to the heart. The SV is used only in exceptional cases, as the risk of pneumothorax is increased. In addition, occlusion of the SV should be avoided, as this would worsen the conditions for successful creation of a hemodialysis shunt on the ipsilateral arm.
b) **Incorrect.** Discharge with a Shaldon catheter is contraindicated because it is not fixed and can easily become dislodged, potentially causing severe bleeding complications. Furthermore, the Shaldon catheter does not have a cuff and the risk of infection is significantly increased. For this reason, outpatient catheter dialysis to bridge the maturation phase of a dialysis shunt is usually performed via a Demers catheter, which is also made of polyurethane or silicone and implanted via the IJV. It is available as a single-, double-, or triple-lumen catheter and also has a so-called Dacron cuff. The

Demers catheter is brought out percutaneously infraclavicularly, and the cuff is placed in the subcutaneous tissue just before the exit site. The cuff serves as infection protection, as it makes it difficult or impossible for bacteria to migrate along the catheter. In addition, after the cuff has grown in, catheter dislocations occur less frequently.

c) **Incorrect.** Atrial catheters (Shaldon and Demers), which are primarily implanted for hemodialysis therapy, do have a larger lumen than central venous catheters (CVCs). This is because CVCs are primarily used for infusion therapy, where flow volume is less important. The diameter of a classic atrial catheter is 15 French (5 mm), allowing flow rates of 300–500 ml/min. Other important differences are that the Demers catheter usually has 2 (or even 3) lumens and a specially configured tip. In single-lumen catheters, the tip is shaped like a fish mouth to prevent it from suctioning onto the vessel wall and causing catheter dysfunction. In double-lumen catheters, the arterial and venous limbs are separated over several centimeters at the tip, referred to as "split." An example is the HemoSplit® catheter from Bard.

d) **Incorrect.** Placement of a Demers catheter should be strictly indicated, as the rate of serious complications (dysfunction, infection, thrombosis of central veins) is not uncommon and should be taken seriously. The complication rate for atrial catheters is 3–4 times higher than for native AV fistulas as dialysis access. Therefore, the NKF-KDOQI (National Kidney Foundation-Kidney Disease Outcomes Quality Initiative) recommends that no more than 10% of dialysis patients should be dialyzed via an atrial catheter for longer than 3 months.

e) **Incorrect.** In Germany, 80% of patients with end-stage renal disease can be dialyzed via a native fistula, and only 20% require an atrial catheter. The most common reason for an atrial catheter is the late scheduling of AV fistula creation and the fact that the maturation phase is not yet complete. Less commonly, sudden and unexpected progression to end-stage renal disease occurs in previously compensated patients. With 80% mature AV fistulas, Germany leads Europe, which is a quality indicator of good interdisciplinary collaboration and planning. In the USA, only 20% of initial dialysis procedures are performed via a shunt, and 80% via an atrial catheter. Among the shunts, > 50% are synthetic, which brings many disadvantages.

Question

3. Which statements about the Cimino shunt are correct?

a) The so-called Cimino shunt was introduced in 1966 by Michael Brescia, James Cimino, and Kenneth Appel.
b) Before the introduction of the Cimino shunt, the only option was to dialyze via an atrial catheter (Shaldon).
c) The Cimino shunt is a simple, minor operation that should preferably be performed as a training procedure at the beginning of residency.
d) The immediate and early occlusion rate of the Cimino shunt is very low, at about 3–5%.
e) The anastomosis in the Cimino shunt should be performed with absorbable suture material.

Answers

a) **Correct.** The three authors presented the first autologous internal hemodialysis shunt in the New England Journal of Medicine (NEJM), revolutionizing hemodialysis therapy for patients with chronic renal insufficiency. This is an arteriovenous anastomosis between the cephalic vein and the radial artery at the level of the wrist.
b) **Incorrect.** Before the introduction of the autologous arteriovenous fistula (AVF), dialysis was primarily performed via external glass (since 1924) or Teflon cannulas (Scribner shunt, since 1960), which was only possible for a limited time. The cannulas were inserted into suitable veins and arteries and fixed to the skin surface. Their durability was only a few weeks, and the access vessels could no longer be used afterward. When all available vessels were exhausted, therapy had to be discontinued and the patient died.
c) **Incorrect.** Although the Cimino shunt is a relatively short procedure (30–60 min), it is quite demanding. It must also be considered that affected patients depend on the reliable and prompt functionality of this vascular access for survival.
d) **Incorrect.** The rate is about 30–50%, which is also the main criticism of this access. This can be explained by the small vessel diameters and the resulting lower blood flow. Nevertheless, especially in young people, the AVF should be created as distally as possible to preserve veins and puncture sites.

e) **Correct.** The advantage of absorbable suture material is that the anastomosis can and should widen over time to increase blood flow. The risk of an anastomotic aneurysm is very low and can be neglected in the Cimino shunt.

Question

4. Which statements about upper arm shunts are correct?

a) The Graz fistula at the level of the elbow is a native autologous fistula.
b) The basilic vein shunt is also one of the native hemodialysis shunts.
c) The PTFE loop shunt in the forearm should generally be preferred over a basilic vein shunt.
d) A PTFE straight shunt can be created if the arterial inflow is suitable but the vein calibers are insufficient.
e) The Appel shunt is a native (autologous) upper arm shunt.

Answers

a) **Correct.** The Graz fistula is a connection between the brachial artery and the cephalic vein or median cubital vein at the level of the elbow. The diameters of the anastomosed vessels are about 3–5 mm. The surgical procedure is relatively simple and short, making it suitable as a training procedure to gain initial experience with anastomosis and the specifics of shunt surgery.
b) **Correct.** The basilic vein shunt is also a native (autologous) upper arm shunt, in which the basilic vein and the brachial (cubital) artery are anastomosed. The diameters of the vessels to be anastomosed are also about 3–5 mm, so this shunt procedure is also suitable for gaining initial experience with anastomosis. However, this type of operation is somewhat more complex than the Graz fistula, especially if the basilic vein is completely mobilized and transposed into the subcutaneous tissue at the time of anastomosis.
c) **Incorrect.** In the PTFE loop shunt, a synthetic graft (usually PTFE standard wall) is anastomosed to the supplying artery and the draining vein and placed in a loop or arc shape in the subcutaneous tissue. This type of shunt should only be indicated if the vascular situation in the arm is unsuitable. The donor vessel is usually the brachial (cubital) artery at the level of the elbow (for a forearm loop shunt) or the axillary artery or proximal brachial artery for an upper arm shunt. In cases where the cephalic vein in the upper arm is too small for shunt creation and a basilic vein shunt is the only available autologous alternative, a PTFE loop shunt in the forearm or elbow can

be created beforehand. Before creating a loop shunt in the axillary region, the native fistula should be preferred if the basilic vein is suitable.

d) **Correct.** In the PTFE straight shunt, the arterial and venous connections are at different levels of the limb. The reasons are usually unsuitable donor or recipient vessels. If the veins are unsuitable, the venous connection is central and the arterial is distal. Conversely, if there are arterial inflow problems, the arterial anastomosis is central and the venous is distal. If both anastomoses are at the same level, the distance is too short and a loop configuration is usually indicated to provide sufficient puncture length.

e) **Incorrect.** Brescia, Cimino, and Appel developed and successfully established the arteriovenous hemodialysis fistula named after them in 1966 (Cimino clearly stood out or prevailed here). However, this is a forearm shunt, the anastomosis between the radial artery and the cephalic vein at the level of the wrist.

Question

5. Which statements regarding the nomenclature of upper arm shunts are correct?

a) The draining vein should always be specified.

b) For alloplastic shunts, the diameter and wall thickness of the material used should always be specified.

c) If available, eponyms (e.g., Graz fistula) should be given for the shunt.

d) When specifying the location of stenoses, occlusions, or aneurysms, proximal = closer to the body and distal = farther from the body, even for AVFs.

e) When creating a basilic vein fistula in the upper arm, the vein is always immediately transposed into the subcutaneous tissue and does not need to be specified separately.

Answers

a) **Correct.** The supplying artery is regularly the brachial artery as the only upper arm artery; the draining veins can be the cephalic vein ("cephalic shunt") or the basilic vein (basilic shunt).

b) **Correct.** These are usually 6–8 mm diameter polytetrafluoroethylene (PTFE) grafts without external ring reinforcement, but with greater wall thickness (standard wall) compared to prostheses used for bypass surgery (thin wall). This is due to the regular puncturing of the shunt prosthesis and the associated increased stress.

c) **Incorrect.** Eponyms should be avoided if possible, as they are not universally known and can lead to confusion or lack of information. The only commonly used eponym is the "Cimino shunt," which refers to the typical anastomosis of the radial artery to the cephalic vein at the level of the wrist.
d) **Incorrect.** For AVFs, proximal should uniformly be equated with "close to the anastomosis," and distal with "far from the anastomosis." Thus, as a rule, proximal = farther from the body and distal = closer to the body. Since this nomenclature is not used consistently, misunderstandings between nephrologists and vascular surgeons are common in clinical practice.
e) **Incorrect.** For the basilic vein fistula, there are two options: either the vein is transposed into the subcutaneous tissue at the time of anastomosis with the brachial artery, or this is done in a second procedure. The disadvantage of the single-stage approach is that the vein must be exposed from the elbow to the axilla, which prolongs the operation time. In addition, it can sometimes be more difficult to perform the procedure under regional anesthesia. Clear advantages, however, are that the medial antebrachial cutaneous nerve, which regularly crosses the basilic vein in the upper arm, is not transected but rather transposed under the distally divided vein, and the shunt can be punctured after 4–6 weeks without another operation.

Question

6. Which statements about native upper arm shunts are correct?

a) The cephalic vein is usually larger in diameter and therefore better suited.
b) The basilic vein lies deeper than the cephalic vein and must regularly be transposed into the subcutaneous tissue.
c) The basilic vein often develops stenoses at the junction with the axillary vein.
d) After the maturation phase, the basilic vein often has a significantly higher flow volume, with the risk of right heart strain and/or steal syndrome.
e) The location of the cephalic vein (lateral-radial) makes it easier and more comfortable for both the patient and the person performing the puncture.

Answers

a) **Incorrect.** The cephalic vein is generally smaller in diameter than the basilic vein. Typical diameters of the cephalic vein are between 3–6 mm, while those of the basilic vein are between 5–8 mm or more.

b) **Correct.** The basilic vein lies subfascially at a depth of often > 10 mm from the skin surface, compared to the cephalic vein. Since the distance to the skin should be < 6 mm to allow puncture and reduce complications, the basilic vein must regularly be dissected along its entire length and transposed into the subcutaneous tissue. This is rarely necessary for the cephalic vein, so the skin incision and access trauma are much shorter and less severe for the latter.
c) **Incorrect.** The basilic vein usually joins the axillary vein at an acute angle, and stenosis is rare here. It is different at the junction of the cephalic vein, which often joins the axillary vein at a right angle or even in a curved, obtuse angle (so-called cephalic arch), making stenosis much more common.
d) **Correct.** Since the basilic vein is generally larger in diameter than the cephalic vein, it often has significantly higher flow volumes after the maturation phase and over time, often 1.5–2.5 L. This must be taken into account during surgical planning and shunt evaluation, especially in patients with pre-existing cardiac disease. Otherwise, acute right heart strain with decompensation is a serious complication.
e) **Correct.** Pain sensitivity on the lateral upper arm is usually less pronounced than on the medial-ulnar side, so the puncture procedure is perceived as less painful. Also, stable placement of the puncture cannulas during the several-hour hemodialysis session is much easier along the natural course of the cephalic vein than with the medially located basilic vein.

Question

7. Which statements about hemodialysis shunts with special indications are correct?

a) The so-called HeRO® shunt can be implanted in cases of central stenosis.
b) The central portion of the HeRO® shunt can no longer be explanted.
c) The so-called Collier shunt is a good alternative to the upper arm shunt.
d) In cases of high surgical risk, an interventional shunt creation should be performed.
e) In interventional shunt creation, a connection is typically made between the radial artery and the cephalic vein in the distal forearm.

Answers

a) **Correct.** The abbreviation HeRO® stands for Hemodialysis Reliable Outflow, which ensures reliable venous outflow. It can be implanted as a last resort in cases of central stenoses; the principle is as follows: the shunt consists of a central component containing nitinol, which is placed under fluoroscopic guidance across the stenoses of the subclavian or brachiocephalic vein. This component is then connected via a special connector to the peripheral PTFE segment, which is anastomosed to the supplying artery or has already been anastomosed beforehand.

b) **Incorrect.** The central component of the HeRO® shunt can be explanted just like an atrial catheter. This is particularly indicated in cases of dysfunction or infection and is usually possible without difficulty.

c) **Incorrect.** The Collier shunt is extremely rarely created and is not an equivalent alternative to an extremity shunt. It is a PTFE shunt that is anastomosed on one side to the subclavian artery, then tunneled subcutaneously like a chain below the jugular notch across the chest to the opposite side, where it is anastomosed to the subclavian vein. The indication for this shunt is comparable to that for the HeRO® shunt—an ipsilateral venous outflow problem.

d) **Incorrect.** In principle, interventional shunt creation is possible; however, this is an alternative to the classic surgically created arteriovenous fistula. The patient's general condition and surgical fitness are not decisive for the indication or the choice between surgical or interventional approach. Both procedures are usually performed under local anesthesia.

e) **Incorrect.** With a special device, EndoAVF® from Ellipsys® (part of Medtronic), the median cubital vein and cubital artery are punctured, a wire is inserted (which then lies in both artery and vein), and the device is introduced over this wire. Its tip is then placed at the connection between artery and vein, these are drawn together, and a short application of current (about 1 s) creates the fistula. The subsequent maturation phase is equivalent to that after surgical fistula creation.

Question

8. Which statements about interventional-radiological shunt creation are correct?

a) Interventional creation of hemodialysis shunts is better suited for children than open surgical creation.

b) The endovascular creation of hemodialysis shunts was developed at about the same time as the EVAR procedure.

c) There is only one device currently available on the market that is approved for endovascular creation of hemodialysis access.
d) The principle of endovascular creation of hemodialysis shunts is the formation of a fistula by perforation and stent placement at the anastomosis site.
e) If the vascular situation at the distal forearm is good, creation of a Cimino shunt should be preferred.

Answers

a) **Incorrect.** There is currently no experience with endovascular shunt creation in children, as the available devices are not approved for pediatric use.
b) **Incorrect.** Endovascular treatment of aortic aneurysms was first performed in 1996 and has been continuously developed since then. In contrast, endovascular creation of hemodialysis shunts has only been performed since 2016, so further developments are still awaited. In particular, long-term results and data are currently not yet available.
c) **Incorrect.** There are currently two different devices from two manufacturers that are approved for endovascular creation of hemodialysis shunts. These are the WavelinQ® EndoAVF system from TVA Medical/Becton Dickinson and Ellipsys® from Medtronic.
d) **Incorrect.** The principle is to create a connection between artery and vein using electrical current or radiofrequency. With the two currently available systems, WavelinQ® EndoAVF and Ellipsys®, the connection between artery and vein is created percutaneously under catheter guidance, but the mechanisms differ:
   I. WavelinQ® EndoAVF: Here, two magnetic catheters are introduced, one via the artery and one via the vein. A radiofrequency generator is then used to create the connection once the two catheters are positioned side by side at the planned anastomosis site.
   II. Ellipsys® from Medtronic: The principle is different; here, the fistula is created via a catheter introduced through the vein. Perforation is then made into the artery, and a special mechanism at the catheter tip closes it. This draws the artery and vein together, and a pulse of current is used to create the fistula.
e) **Correct.** If the vascular situation at the distal forearm is good, surgical creation of an arteriovenous fistula at the wrist, i.e., a Cimino shunt, is still recommended. With endovascular procedures, the arteriovenous fistula is generally created at the level of the elbow; more distal application is not yet established.

Question

9. Which statements about alloplastic materials in hemodialysis shunts are correct?

a) Polytetrafluoroethylene (PTFE) is approved as standard wall (SW) and thin wall (TW) prostheses for hemodialysis shunts.
b) Standard wall (SW) PTFE prostheses are preferable to thin wall (TW) prostheses for dialysis shunts.
c) Standard wall (SW) PTFE prostheses can be punctured earlier than thin wall (TW) prostheses.
d) There are also PTFE prostheses that can be punctured within a few hours after shunt creation.
e) PTFE prostheses for hemodialysis shunts should have a diameter of at least 8 mm to avoid stenoses.

Answers

a) **Correct.** Both types of prostheses are available from WL Gore and are approved for use in synthetic shunt creation. Both have a diameter of 6 mm; the wall thickness is 0.6 mm for SW prostheses and 0.3–0.4 mm for TW prostheses.
b) **Correct.** There are studies showing that the patency rates of SW prostheses are significantly better than those of TW prostheses, regarding both primary and secondary as well as cumulative patency.[1] However, the infection rate and aneurysm formation were comparable.
c) **Incorrect.** Both SW and TW prostheses should not be punctured earlier than 4–6 weeks after shunt implantation. Otherwise, the risk of bleeding, dysfunction, early occlusion, and infection is increased. For alloplastic shunts, the decisive factor is not the wall thickness of the prosthesis, but its integration into the soft tissue, i.e., tissue ingrowth. This reduces the risk of periprosthetic hematoma formation during the healing period, which becomes minimal after 4–6 weeks.

[1] Lenz BJ, Veldenz HC, Dennis JW, Khansarinia S, Atteberry LR. A three-year follow-up on standard versus thin wall ePTFE grafts for hemodialysis. J Vasc Surg. 1998 Sep;28(3):464–70; discussion 470. https://doi.org/10.1016/s0741-5214(98)70132-6. PMID: 9737456.

d) **Correct.** There are also early-puncturable prostheses (e.g., Acuseal® from WL Gore) that can be punctured within 24–48 hours after shunt creation. There have even been reports of this prosthesis type being used successfully and without complications as early as 2 hours after placement. The principle is an additional elastomer layer between the outer and inner PTFE membranes, which acts as a seal. However, special puncture needles must be used, which must be inserted at an angle and against the direction of blood flow.

e) **Incorrect.** PTFE prostheses for hemodialysis shunts are usually the same as those used for peripheral bypasses and are preferably used in diameters of 6 mm. These 6 mm prostheses are available in standard wall (SW) configuration with a wall thickness of 0.6 mm and in thin wall (TW) configuration with wall thicknesses of 0.3–0.4 mm. In addition, a conically configured SW-PTFE prosthesis was developed primarily for use in dialysis shunt creation, with different diameters at each end (4 mm and 7 mm). The 7 mm end is anastomosed to the venous (outflow) end of the shunt, the 4 mm end to the arterial (inflow) anastomosis. This is intended to reduce the risk of stenosis at the venous anastomosis, a common cause of shunt occlusion. The reduction of the diameter at the arterial anastomosis to 4 mm aims to minimize the risk of a "high-flow" situation.

Question

10. Which statements about surgical shunt revisions are correct?

a) For basilic vein shunts, subcutaneous transposition of the vein should always be performed in two stages.

b) If there are multiple aneurysms of the shunt vein, all should be treated in a single operation to spare the patient repeated surgeries.

c) Only autologous material should be used for surgical shunt revisions.

d) For shunt revisions using synthetic material, thicker-walled PTFE prostheses are recommended.

e) Xenogeneic replacement in hemodialysis shunts is not approved.

Answers

a) **Incorrect.** It is possible to initially anastomose the basilic vein only distally to the brachial artery and leave it proximally in situ. However, since the vein is usually too deep, it must be transposed from the subfascial area to beneath the skin before the first puncture. This can be done during a second operation. However, it is also quite possible to do this directly during the initial anastomosis procedure. The advantage is that the patient does not need a second operation, and the medial brachial cutaneous nerve, which crosses the basilic vein in the upper arm, must be transected during the two-stage procedure. With direct transposition of the vein during the initial procedure, the vein is ligated distally, completely mobilized, and placed over the nerve, thus preserving it. Transection of the nerve leads to sensory disturbances in the medial upper arm and proximal forearm.

b) **Incorrect.** In principle, a compromise should be reached between the extent of the procedure and the available or remaining puncture segment. If several consecutive aneurysms are perfused and not occluded, multiple revisions should be performed. For example, first resect the aneurysms near the anastomosis with a remaining puncture segment above; after 6–8 weeks, when the wound has healed, treat the remaining aneurysm(s). If necessary, the approach can be extended to more than two surgical sessions. If the entire altered shunt vein is revised in one session, there may be no puncture segment left, and an atrial catheter may have to be placed. This should always be avoided if possible.

c) **Incorrect.** The main goal of surgical shunt revisions is to correct stenoses, occlusions, aneurysms, or infections. Other, less common reasons include high-flow shunts with or without additional steal phenomenon, as well as closure in the case of a functioning transplant kidney. In clinical practice, urgent shunt revisions for acute occlusions make up the majority of indications. Most often, these are occlusions due to pre-existing stenoses. In addition to thrombectomy, reconstruction or replacement of stenotic areas may be necessary, usually using synthetic material. The aim is to preserve available vein material for possible future shunt creation.

d) **Correct.** For primary creation of synthetic shunts and surgical shunt revisions, so-called “standard wall prostheses” have proven effective. Compared to “thin wall prostheses,” which are used for peripheral bypasses, these have a thicker and thus more puncture-resistant wall.

e) **Incorrect.** Xenogeneic replacement of stenotic or aneurysmal hemodialysis shunts can also be performed using bovine material (e.g., in the form of Xenosure® patches or the Omniflow-II prosthesis® from LeMaitre, which is already available as a loop). However, it should be noted that degeneration occurs more frequently, which may necessitate further revisions.

Question

11. Which statements about hemodialysis via atrial catheters are correct?

a) Dialysis via an atrial catheter has been successfully introduced since 1930.
b) The Shaldon catheter can be implanted via the jugular, subclavian, or femoral vein.
c) A Shaldon catheter can remain in place for several weeks or months, especially to bridge the maturation phase of a shunt if necessary.
d) When creating a new hemodialysis shunt, an atrial catheter should be generously implanted to allow dialysis via the Demers catheter during the shunt's maturation phase if needed.
e) There are different catheter tip designs to best separate the venous and arterial limbs.

Answers

a) **Incorrect.** The first atrial catheter for acute dialysis was invented by Shaldon in 1961 and named after him. In 1970, the Demers catheter was introduced, which, unlike the Shaldon catheter, had a so-called cuff that grows into the tissue and thus serves as a bacterial filter or barrier. As a result, the Demers catheter became infected much less frequently and could remain in place for several months, sometimes even years.
b) **Correct.** Large-bore central venous catheters used for hemodialysis can be implanted via the internal and external jugular veins, the subclavian vein, or, in exceptional cases, the femoral vein. Due to its good accessibility, the internal jugular vein is most commonly used, especially since this approach can be performed by puncture and is now often carried out by dialysis physicians themselves.
c) **Incorrect.** The Shaldon catheter is intended only for short-term hemodialysis; discharge to the home environment is not permitted with a Shaldon catheter in place. This is because the catheter is not secured, so it can dislocate and lead to potentially fatal bleeding complications. Furthermore, the risk of infection is significantly higher with the Shaldon catheter than with the Demers, which also argues against prolonged use. The infection protection of the Demers is due to the obligatory felt cuff, which is placed in the subcutaneous tissue and grows in. This significantly reduces the risk of bacterial colonization and thus catheter infection.

d) **Incorrect.** Ideally, the shunt is created in the pre-terminal stage to allow sufficient time for the arteriovenous fistula to mature. Therefore, good planning by nephrologists and timely referral of these patients to vascular surgeons is essential and a quality marker of interdisciplinary collaboration. Placement of an atrial catheter should only be done in exceptional cases, as the risk of catheter infection, thrombosis, or other complications in the central veins should be avoided.
e) **Correct.** To separate recirculated and non-recirculated blood at the catheter tip and thus make hemodialysis as effective as possible, different catheter tip designs have been developed. These include simple, pointed catheters (pointed), which are easy to implant but have a high recirculation rate. They are now also available with side holes (multiperforated). There are also split tips, which can be more difficult to implant, and offset openings (step tip, usually 2.5 cm between the openings of the arterial and venous limbs). Finally, there are symmetrically coiled tips (as in the Palindrome™ series from Medtronic).

Question

12. Which statements about the Allen test are correct?

a) The Allen test is used before creation of Cimino shunts.
b) The Allen test is only used in vascular surgery.
c) In the Allen test, the radial and ulnar arteries are manually compressed until the hand turns white (ischemia), and then released individually.
d) Normally, it takes < 5 s for the hand to become pink again.
e) If the hand is not adequately reperfused until > 5 s later, the Allen test is negative.

Answers

a) **Correct.** The Allen test is used before creation of hemodialysis shunts in the forearm, especially Cimino shunts. It tests hand perfusion and the functionality of collaterals. It also assesses whether perfusion via the ulnar artery is sufficient to avoid ischemia after anastomosis to the radial artery.
b) **Incorrect.** Although the Allen test is most often associated with shunt surgery and was first described and used there, it tests the functionality of the radial and ulnar arteries regarding hand perfusion. However, there are other applications, such as:

I. Intensive care medicine: before placement of an arterial line ("artery") at the wrist
II. Plastic surgery: before creation of a radial forearm flap
III. Cardiology: before transradial cardiac catheterization
IV. Cardiac surgery: before harvesting the radial artery as a graft for coronary bypasses

c) **Correct.** The purpose of the Allen test is to assess hand perfusion, especially the functionality of the artery (usually the ulnar artery) that will not be anastomosed to the shunt vein. When both arteries are compressed above systolic pressure, ischemia (whitening) occurs; after releasing each artery individually, their contribution to perfusion can be tested. If the hand quickly becomes pink again after releasing the ulnar artery, perfusion via this artery is sufficient and there is no contraindication to anastomosis to the radial artery.
d) **Correct.** After whitening of the hand and selective release of the arteries, perfusion normally returns to normal within less than 5 s. If the hand only returns to normal color after more than 5 s, this indicates advanced arteriosclerosis or stenosis.
e) **Incorrect.** The Allen test is negative if reperfusion occurs quickly, i.e., within < 5 s after release of the artery being tested. If the artery is stenosed and reperfusion takes longer than 5–7 s, the test is positive. In summary, as a mnemonic: a **p**ositive Allen test is **p**athological and a poor result for perfusion.

Question

13. Which statements about puncture techniques for a hemodialysis shunt are correct?

a) There are five common puncture techniques for hemodialysis shunts.
b) In principle, the rope ladder puncture technique should be preferred.
c) Buttonhole puncture of a hemodialysis shunt is now obsolete.
d) With area puncture, stenoses and hypoplastic venous segments can be gradually dilated.
e) A puncture aneurysm of a hemodialysis shunt is a sign of insufficient care in the choice of puncture technique.

Answers

a) **Incorrect.** Three puncture techniques for dialysis shunts are more commonly used in clinical practice:
   I. Rope ladder,
   II. Area, and
   III. Buttonhole puncture

b) **Incorrect.** In the rope ladder technique, the shunt vein is punctured along its entire length, essentially from top to bottom. This requires a precise scheme that must be followed for each dialysis cycle, ensuring a new puncture site outside the previous one each time.
   The advantage of the rope ladder technique is the use of the entire vein segment, thereby promoting the durability and lifespan of the hemodialysis shunt. Rope ladder puncture is therefore recommended for unremarkable and functional shunts without stenoses or aneurysms.

c) **Incorrect.** The principle of the buttonhole technique is that the shunt vein is punctured at one (or a few) sites in exactly the same way each time (same needle gauge, same puncture angle, precisely the same spot). This creates a puncture channel that is closed by a thrombus after removal of the cannula and temporary compression. The advantage of this technique is reduced pain during puncture, which is why it is regularly recommended and often successfully used, especially in younger or very pain-sensitive patients.

d) **Correct.** In area puncture, the shunt vein is punctured in specific segments. After removal of the cannula, a small local thrombus forms in the puncture channel, sealing the puncture. Subsequently, the thrombus is organized into scar tissue, resulting in new tissue formation. This is also called remodeling. Due to this remodeling, each puncture leads to a slight tissue expansion at the puncture site, which can gradually enlarge hypoplastic segments.

e) **Incorrect.** Puncture aneurysm of a hemodialysis shunt is a very common complication and can occur with all common puncture techniques. It occurs least frequently with the buttonhole technique, but cannot be ruled out even then. Other causes of a puncture aneurysm include stenoses along the vein, with aneurysms typically occurring downstream.

Question

14. Which statements about acute shunt occlusion are correct?

a) A hemodialysis shunt occludes on average 2–3 times per year.
b) The most common cause of acute shunt occlusion is thrombosis due to dehydration.
c) Aneurysms lead to a "high volume" shunt, but not to occlusion.
d) An acute shunt occlusion almost always necessitates placement of an atrial catheter.
e) Acute shunt occlusions must be treated surgically; radiological-interventional therapy is not an option here.

Answers

a) **Correct.** The most common complication of a hemodialysis shunt is acute occlusion. Statistically, this occurs 2–3 times per year, which is related to the inherent stress on this vascular access. The dialysis shunt is the only vascular surgical "reconstruction" that is regularly punctured and compressed. No other bypass is subjected to such strain and is at the same time as vital as the dialysis shunt.
b) **Incorrect.** The most common cause of acute shunt occlusion is stenoses, aneurysms, or both along the shunt vein. These create passage obstructions, which typically lead to thrombotic occlusion. In prosthetic shunts, stenoses are typically found at the prosthetic-venous anastomosis.
c) **Incorrect.** Aneurysms, after stenoses, are also a common cause of shunt occlusions, and often both are present in combination. Since stenoses develop over time, aneurysms of the shunt vein frequently occur downstream. This is most likely due to post-stenotic turbulence.
d) **Incorrect.** Ideally, the shunt can and should be reopened surgically or interventionally as quickly as possible to restore its use for hemodialysis. The operating surgeon should therefore suspect or localize the underlying cause before making the skin incision, in order to keep the access to the shunt vein as small as possible. The goal should be to preserve as much of the puncture segment as possible.
e) **Incorrect.** Acute shunt occlusions can also be successfully treated interventionally. Even prolonged lysis therapy ("long-term lysis with rt-PA") lasting several hours (even overnight) with percutaneous angioplasty of

underlying, unmasked stenoses is practiced in many hospitals. The advantages of these procedures are shorter patient stays (sometimes outpatient), the use of local anesthesia without anesthesia-related complications or contraindications in hyperkalemia, avoidance of skin incisions, and avoidance of foreign materials (prosthetic shunts).

Question

15. Which statements about shunt aneurysms are correct?

a) Shunt aneurysms are a surgically induced complication of hemodialysis shunts.
b) Shunt aneurysms must be treated surgically at an early stage.
c) Shunt aneurysms are almost exclusively false aneurysms.
d) Shunt aneurysms should be excluded, as with aortic aneurysms, by open or endovascular means.
e) The so-called buttonhole technique leads to shunt aneurysms less frequently than the rope ladder technique.

Answers

a) **Incorrect.** Shunt aneurysms are a common complication of both autologous and alloplastic hemodialysis accesses. They usually arise due to multiple punctures, especially with area and buttonhole techniques. Scar tissue forms, which is less resistant than the original vessel wall, typically resulting in aneurysms. However, aneurysms can also occur at the anastomosis of alloplastic shunts and due to infection.
b) **Incorrect.** In principle, shunt aneurysms only need to be treated surgically if complications arise. Typical surgical indications are:
   I. Infections and exposed PTFE segments
   II. High-flow situation with steal syndrome and/or cardiac strain
   III. Shunt dysfunction due to upstream stenoses or
   IV. Shunt thromboses
   V. progressively enlarging false aneurysms with tension-related skin lesions

   There is no elective surgical indication based on diameter alone.
c) **Incorrect.** Shunt aneurysms are indeed also puncture aneurysms, i.e., false aneurysms. However, true aneurysms, which also arise from the regularly necessary punctures, are more common. In this case, the entire vessel wall bulges out due to puncture-related scarring changes. Unlike false aneu-

rysms in arteries, puncture aneurysms of hemodialysis shunts rarely present as a "pulsating hematoma."

d) **Incorrect.** The preferred surgical approach, which is often favored and yields good results, is removal of thrombi, aneurysm plication or resection, and end-to-end anastomosis. Plication of the aneurysm with simultaneous autologous patch plasty of adjacent (usually upstream) stenoses has also proven effective. The use of prosthetic material as an interposition graft should be avoided if possible, especially in infection-related aneurysms.
e) **Correct.** According to current studies, the buttonhole technique leads to the formation of shunt aneurysms significantly less often than the rope ladder technique. The principle of the buttonhole technique is to puncture the shunt at the same site each time, initially with a sharp needle, later with a blunt one. The blunt needle can be used once the puncture channel has stabilized. This technique is also associated with less pain for patients. However, a disadvantage of the buttonhole technique appears to be an increased risk of infection, which is why it should be avoided in PTFE shunts if possible. In the rope ladder technique, the shunt is always punctured at a different site, following a fixed scheme resembling a rope ladder.

Question

16. Which statements about infection of a dialysis shunt are correct?

a) Infection of an autologous hemodialysis shunt is very rare.
b) An infected native upper arm shunt usually requires surgical treatment.
c) Shunt infections account for < 1% of inpatient dialysis shunt complications.
d) Bioprostheses (e.g., umbilical veins) are infected significantly less often than PTFE prostheses.
e) An anechoic fluid collection around a PTFE prosthetic shunt is often due to infection.

Answers

a) **Correct.** Infection of shunts is overall a rare complication, accounting for less than 10% of complications. Infection of autologous shunts is much less common than that of alloplastic accesses, accounting for < 1% of all complications. In other words: infection of a prosthetic shunt is 3 to 5 times more common than that of native shunts, which is a significant advantage of these dialysis accesses.

b) **Incorrect.** An infected autologous shunt in the upper arm, e.g., due to an infected aneurysm, can usually be treated conservatively. With antiseptic local therapy using moist, cooling, and disinfecting dressings and antibiotics, autologous shunt infections can almost always be successfully managed. The situation is different with PTFE shunts. In the vast majority of cases, these must be surgically revised and even explanted if infected. Infected prosthetic shunts are a rare but very serious complication. This is further complicated by the fact that multimorbid patients with end-stage renal disease usually have a weakened immune system and are susceptible to local and especially systemic infections.

c) **Incorrect.** Shunt infections are indeed very rare and, especially in native fistulas, account for a very small proportion (< 1%) of shunt complications. Nevertheless, the proportion of dialysis shunt complications requiring inpatient treatment is higher, accounting for about 10% in Germany. This is partly because more common complications such as acute shunt occlusion and dysfunction can often be treated on an outpatient basis, whereas shunt infection almost always requires inpatient treatment. In the USA, the proportion of shunt infections among inpatient cases of hemodialysis shunt complications is even higher, at about 25%. One reason for this may be the significantly higher number of patients receiving prosthetic shunts.

d) **Incorrect.** Bioprostheses (e.g., umbilical veins) were once preferred as vascular substitutes for dialysis shunts, but showed a significantly increased infection rate of up to 25%. By comparison: prosthetic shunts have an infection rate of about 5–10%, native shunts < 5%. Consequently, bioprostheses in the form of umbilical veins have not become established as substitutes for dialysis shunts. Increased hematoma formation and aneurysms were suspected as reasons for the higher infection rate.

e) **Incorrect.** A fluid collection around a PTFE shunt prosthesis is often due to infection, but sterile perigraft reactions can also be the cause. In a perigraft reaction, a fluid collection forms around an alloplastic prosthesis, with PTFE being affected much more frequently than, for example, Dacron. The fluid is almost always sterile and often has a gelatinous consistency. A graft-versus-host reaction is suspected as the cause. This reaction most commonly occurs within the first weeks after implantation, but can persist for years. An echo-poor or anechoic fluid formation around a PTFE prosthesis in completely unremarkable soft tissue without any signs of inflammation is usually a perigraft reaction and can almost always be successfully treated conservatively.

Question

17. Which statements about steal syndrome after creation of a dialysis shunt are correct?

a) This involves a flow reversal in the artery distal to the arteriovenous anastomosis, resulting in peripheral hypoperfusion.
b) HAIDI is a common complication after creation of Cimino shunts.
c) MILLER banding is a minimally invasive procedure established by the eponymous surgeon for the treatment of steal syndrome in hemodialysis shunts.
d) Every steal syndrome of a dialysis shunt should be treated surgically or interventionally.
e) Banding is the only therapeutic procedure for steal syndrome.

Answers

a) **Incorrect.** Steal syndrome is a peripheral hypoperfusion caused by a flow reversal in the artery supplying the hypoperfused tissue. For example, in subclavian steal syndrome, there is a flow reversal in the vertebral artery due to a stenosis of the subclavian artery proximal to the vertebral origin. In the case of hypoperfusion of the extremity on the shunt arm (usually hand and fingers), often referred to as steal syndrome, there is not a flow reversal in the artery, but rather a significant drop in pressure and thus a perfusion deficit. The correct term should therefore be HAIDI (hemodialysis access induced distal ischemia). However, this term has not yet become established in clinical practice.
b) **Incorrect.** HAIDI is a rare complication after creation of hemodialysis shunts and occurs much more frequently in upper arm than in forearm shunts. In Cimino shunts, this complication is extremely rare, especially if the Allen test was consistently performed preoperatively and yielded unremarkable findings.
c) **Correct.** MILLER banding is a minimally invasive endoluminal-assisted surgical procedure in which a balloon is percutaneously placed in the anastomosis or outflow shunt vein and inflated to a predefined diameter. The banding is then performed by placing a strong ligature, either percutaneously or via a small skin incision. The abbreviation MILLER stands for "**M**inimally **I**nvasive **L**imited **L**igation **E**ndoluminal-assisted **R**evision."

What many do not know is that one of the inventors of this procedure was actually named Miller[2].

d) **Incorrect.** Steal syndrome is classified into stages 1–4, which means:
   1. No symptoms, sonographic evidence
   2. Pain on exertion (especially during dialysis)
   3. Pain at rest
   4. Ulcerations

   As with PAD, the indication for further measures is based on the stage. In stages 3 and 4, intervention should be generously indicated, as limb loss is at risk. In stage 1, conservative management is recommended; in stage 2, decisions can be made on an individual basis.

e) **Incorrect.** Banding is certainly the oldest therapeutic procedure. The primary goal is to reduce the diameter and thus the flow in the shunt. However, there are other methods aimed at improving peripheral perfusion. These include, among others:
   - Proximalization of the anastomosis
     - the anastomosis is created more proximally
     - The principle behind this method is the idea that "tapping" a larger-caliber artery has relatively less impact distal to the anastomosis than withdrawing almost the entire flow volume from a small-caliber artery
   - The PAI procedure (proximal arterial inflow)
     - The principle here is that a bypass is sewn from proximal to the anastomosis onto the shunt vein and the original anastomosis is closed
     - Here too, blood for the shunt is drawn from a larger vessel, which, based on experience, leads to fewer ischemic symptoms than with distal anastomoses
   - The RUDI procedure (revision using distal inflow)
     - ultimately, it could also be called DAI (distal arterial inflow)
     - The principle is that a bypass is created from distal to the anastomosis onto the shunt vein and the anastomosis is closed
     - the original arterial pathway for hand perfusion is thus prioritized
   - The DRIL procedure (distal recanalization interval ligation)
     - this is the only procedure in which the native arterial pathway is ligated

[2] Miller GA, Goel N, Friedman A, Khariton A, Jotwani MC, Savransky Y, Khariton K, Arnold WP, Preddie DC. The MILLER banding procedure is an effective method for treating dialysis-associated steal syndrome. Kidney Int. 2010 Feb;77(4):359–66. https://doi.org/10.1038/ki.2009.461.

Question

18. Which statements about ongoing studies on dialysis accesses are correct?

a) The HASE study investigates the impact of sonographic flow measurement during hemodialysis on the patency rates of dialysis shunts.
b) The ACCESS-HD study compares complication rates of AVF and AVG in hemodialysis patients.
c) The DeVA study compares drug eluting balloons (DEB) with standard balloon catheters in the treatment of shunt stenoses.
d) To date, there is no study comparing xenogeneic dialysis shunts (bovine pericardium) with PTFE shunts.
e) The research question of the CITES study is whether central venous thrombosis occurs more frequently after implantation of dialysis catheters via the left IJV than via the right side.

Answers

a) **Correct.** The Hemodialysis Access Surveillance Evaluation (HASE) study investigates the impact of shunt flow measurement during hemodialysis treatment. Using a special program and sensors (HD03 from Transonic) attached to the arterial and venous limbs of the dialysis machine, flow measurements and the degree of recirculation can be regularly documented. The aim is to detect and treat stenoses early to prevent thrombotic shunt occlusions. The patency rates of the "Transonic intervention group" are compared with those receiving standard sonographic or clinical monitoring outside of dialysis at 4-week intervals. At present, the study is not yet complete, and the planned number of patients has not yet been reached.
b) **Incorrect.** The Comparing Catheters to Fistulas in Elderly Patients Starting Hemodialysis (ACCESS HD) study is a multicenter RCT in the USA and Canada, enrolling recently dialysis-dependent patients aged 55 years or older who are initially treated via an atrial catheter. Randomization then assigns patients either to continue dialysis via an atrial catheter or to a second group receiving an arteriovenous shunt as permanent dialysis access. Morbidity and mortality are compared, specifically regarding access-associated complications.
c) **Correct.** The Drug Eluting Balloon Venoplasty in AV Fistula Stenosis (DeVA) study is a multicenter RCT in which shunt stenoses are treated either with a DEB or a standard balloon, and patency rates are compared.

d) **Incorrect.** A single-center study from Baltimore (ClinicalTrials.gov NCT03300024) aims to randomize 100 patients who cannot receive a native shunt into two groups (bovine shunt versus PTFE) and compare patency and complication rates. Infections and soft tissue reactions are of particular interest. Results and publication are expected soon.
e) **Incorrect.** The CITES study investigates whether there is a significant difference in the development of central venous stenosis or thrombosis after implantation of a dialysis catheter via the right IJV compared to the right subclavian vein. It is a multicenter study from Sweden, enrolling 100 patients randomized to receive a catheter subclavian (50 patients) or jugular (50 patients). The background is that data from 1990 to 2000 led to the clinical recommendation to implant dialysis catheters primarily via the IJV rather than the subclavian vein, as thromboses of the subclavian vein were more common at that time. However, materials and implantation techniques have since changed, with ultrasound-guided procedures resulting in fewer venous injuries, and silicone catheters now being used more often than polyurethane. The former are less thrombogenic and more flexible than polyurethane, resulting in a lower risk of thrombosis.

Question

19. Which statements about randomized controlled studies on hemodialysis shunts are correct?

a) The REVISE study investigated whether stent-assisted PTA in synthetic shunts has better patency rates than plain balloon PTA.
b) The PATENCY-1 study investigated whether arteriovenous fistulas (AVF) in the upper arm have better patency rates than arteriovenous grafts (AVG) made of PTFE.
c) To date, there is no randomized study in which end-to-side anastomosis in the creation of an AVF is superior to side-to-side anastomosis.
d) The Kidney Disease Outcomes Quality Initiative (KDOQI) guidelines recommend the following order for AVF selection: 1. radiocephalic, 2. brachiocephalic, 3. brachiobasilic, which has been clearly demonstrated in studies.
e) A randomized study showed that, for hemodialysis shunts in the arm, the GSV as a homologous substitute has fewer infectious complications than PTFE.

Answers

a) **Correct.** The REVISE study is a multicenter study in which patients with synthetic shunts and prior PTA for shunt dysfunction or occlusion received either a stent-PTA (ViaBahn® by WL Gore) or repeat PTA alone to maintain shunt function. Stent-assisted PTA was advantageous in thrombotically occluded shunts, with a significantly better patency rate and fewer interventions over time, whereas there was no difference in cases of shunt dysfunction.

b) **Incorrect.** The PATENCY-1 study investigated whether a human recombinant elastase (vonapanitase) can improve the patency of AVF in dialysis patients. This elastase is thought to dissolve or reduce atherosclerotic plaques in cell cultures and is a major hope for the conservative treatment of patients with atherosclerosis. When used in newly created AVF, it was hoped to achieve better maturation and fewer shunt dysfunctions. However, the primary patency rate showed no significant difference compared to the placebo group, while the secondary patency rate was significantly better in the "vonapanitase" group. The exact mechanisms and reasons for this are still being investigated.

c) **Incorrect.** Most recently, in 2021, there was a randomized single-center study[3], in which end-to-side anastomosis (E-S) was significantly superior to side-to-side anastomosis (S-S) in terms of fistula maturation and functionality: 70% E-S vs. 34% S-S ($p=0.0001$). Consequently, despite the introduction of endovascular techniques, which functionally create an S-S anastomosis, surgical practice continues to recommend E-S anastomosis.

d) **Incorrect.** There is no clear evidence that, in the case of unsuitable vascular conditions in the forearm, a cephalic vein shunt should be preferred over a basilic vein shunt in the upper arm. In a randomized study[4] both shunt types did not differ in either primary or secondary patency rates. The only significant difference was the duration of the surgical procedure, which was significantly longer for the basilic vein shunt. This is because, in

---

[3] ElKassaby M, Elsayed N, Mosaad A, Soliman M. End-to-side versus side-to-side anastomosis with distal vein ligation for arteriovenous fistula creation. Vascular. 2021 Oct;29(5):790–796.

[4] Koksoy C, Demirci RK, Balci D, Solak T, Köse SK. Brachiobasilic versus brachiocephalic arteriovenous fistula: a prospective randomized study. J Vasc Surg. 2009 Jan;49(1):171–177.

a single-stage procedure, the vein must be dissected along its entire length and transposed into the subcutaneous tissue. In the two-stage procedure, which is preferred by some surgeons, the operative times and extent of the access wounds are comparable, but a second operation for subcutaneous transposition of the vein is required for the basilic vein shunt. In summary, there are indeed arguments for preferring the cephalic vein fistula, but not because of better patency rates, rather due to less access trauma and shorter operative times under local or regional anesthesia.

e) **Correct.** In a 2011 study[5] it was shown that infectious complications occurred significantly less frequently when cryopreserved GSV was used as a shunt substitute compared to PTFE prostheses. However, patency rates were comparable. The use of GSV has not become established in clinical practice, which may be due to several reasons, including the better availability and lower cost of PTFE prostheses, as well as the shorter operative time in the case of autologous harvesting and transplantation of the GSV. Not to be neglected is also the strategic "preservation" of the GSV for possible future peripheral or coronary bypass reconstructions, which is not uncommon in this multimorbid patient population with cardiovascular risk factors.

Question

20. Which statements about children requiring dialysis are correct?

a) In children, a Cimino shunt should not be created in the forearm due to the small-caliber vessels.
b) Peritoneal dialysis is contraindicated in children due to the high risk of infection.
c) Kidney transplantation in children can only be performed after the age of 5 years.
d) About 10% of kidney transplants performed annually are in children and adolescents.
e) Since the waiting time for kidney transplantation in children is usually only a few months, a central venous catheter should preferably be used as a dialysis access for bridging.

[5] Mousavi SR, Moatamedi MR, Me Akbari M. Comparing frozen saphenous vein with Gore-tex in vascular access for chronic hemodialysis. Hemodial Int. 2011 Oct;15(4):559–62.

Answers

a) **Incorrect.** The principle also applies to children that the shunt should be placed as distally as possible in order to preserve sufficient proximal vein material for possible future shunt creation. Since children have significantly smaller vessels than adults, the patency rate is lower and the risk of immediate occlusion is higher. Nevertheless, whenever possible, an attempt should be made to create a Cimino shunt. In children weighing less than 20 kg, however, another dialysis modality should be chosen if possible. Ideally, peritoneal dialysis is recommended here, as the risk of complications after placement of an autologous shunt is significantly higher than in older children and adults.

b) **Incorrect.** Children in particular benefit from peritoneal dialysis, as it results in less circulatory strain, the dialysis treatment can take place and be scheduled at home, and regular, uninterrupted school attendance is possible. With adequate training and instruction of patients and parents, the risk of infection is no higher than in adults and is not a contraindication for peritoneal dialysis in children. On the contrary, peritoneal dialysis is even preferred in children.

c) **Incorrect.** As a rule, kidney transplantation in children can be performed from a body weight of 8–10 kg, which is reached by the end of the first to second year of life. Since this usually involves a living donation from relatives, especially the parents, there must be sufficient space in the small pelvis for the adult kidney. In addition, younger children have a higher rate of rejection and complications. Nevertheless, kidney transplantation can be successfully performed well before the age of 5 years.

d) **Correct.** Of the approximately 2000 kidney transplants performed annually, 150–250 are in children. Most of these are living donations, which offer many advantages, especially for children. In particular, the ability to plan living donation and the significant reduction in waiting times shortens the suffering of young patients and reduces the resulting sequelae caused by renal insufficiency and dialysis therapy.

e) **Incorrect.** Firstly, even in children, the average waiting time for kidney transplantation is 24 months or longer, especially if a cadaveric kidney is involved. Furthermore, as with adults, but especially in children, catheter dialysis should be avoided whenever possible. This is particularly due to possible complications such as infections, thrombosis of the access vessels, and thus deterioration of the vascular situation for future shunt creation. The complication rate of central venous catheters for hemodialysis is up to

60 times higher than that of arteriovenous shunts, and the infection rate is about 10 times higher than that of arteriovenous grafts. According to guideline recommendations, a maximum of 10% of dialysis patients should be dialyzed permanently via a catheter. This applies not only to adults but also to pediatric patients. However, the reality is different: 60–70% of children are dialyzed via a catheter.

8 Venous Diseases

Question

1. Which statements about the epidemiology of venous thromboses are correct?

a) The incidence of deep vein thrombosis is 1–2/1000/year.
b) The greatest risk factor for the development of DVT is the combination of nicotine abuse and the use of contraceptives.
c) In Europe, more people die from pulmonary embolism than from breast and prostate cancer, HIV/AIDS, and traffic accidents combined.
d) Within 5 years, approximately 30% of patients with DVT experience a recurrent thrombosis.
e) DVT and pulmonary embolism can be the first sign of a malignant disease.

Answers

a) **Correct.** The annual incidence of venous thromboembolism, which includes deep vein thrombosis and pulmonary embolism, remains relatively high despite significant advances in anticoagulation therapy and has remained unchanged over the years at around 0.1–0.3% annually.
b) **Incorrect.** The most significant influence and risk factor for the development of DVT is age. The annual incidence of DVT is age-dependent:
   I. in those under 20 years: 1/10,000
   II. in adults aged 20–60 years: 1/1000
   III. in those aged 60 years: 1–3/100

S. Regus, *Vascular Surgery: Questions and Answers*,
https://doi.org/10.1007/978-3-662-73387-5_8

Thus, age is the greatest and at the same time non-modifiable risk factor for the development of DVT.

c) **Correct.** According to study results (VITAE study from 2007), more than 1 million people in Europe (Germany, France, Italy, England, Spain, and Portugal) develop venous thromboembolism each year, of which approximately 400,000 are fatal. This has significant implications for the healthcare system and treating physicians, especially since the majority of DVTs and pulmonary embolisms (PE) occur during or in the immediate temporal context of a hospital stay.
d) **Incorrect.** The risk of recurrent thrombosis is approximately 30% after 10 years; independent risk factors include age, obesity, nicotine abuse and contraception, malignant diseases, and immobility.
e) **Correct.** Pulmonary embolisms (PE) occur more frequently in patients with underlying malignant diseases and are often fulminant. PE is among the most common causes of death in cancer patients. Patients with pancreatic and ovarian carcinomas are particularly at risk of developing venous complications.

Question

2. Which statements about the development of venous thromboses are correct?

a) In the vast majority of cases, the veins of the lower extremity are affected.
b) The main risk factor for the development of thrombosis is female sex.
c) Virchow's triad is only important in arterial thromboses and is negligible in venous ones.
d) The Wells score is helpful in the diagnosis of venous thromboses and is based on the typical etiology and pathogenesis of thromboses.
e) Immobility is the main risk factor for thromboses, which is why they are an absolute rarity in athletes.

Answers

a) **Correct.** In over 90% of cases, the inferior vena cava (IVC) as well as the superficial and deep veins of the lower extremities are affected. This is due to the natural burden of gravity in upright humans and the strain during sedentary activities.

b) **Incorrect.** The main risk factor is age. With increasing age, the annual incidence of deep vein thrombosis (DVT) increases:
   1. up to age 20: 1/100,000
   2. ages 20–40: 1/10,000
   3. ages 40–60: 1/1000
   4. > 60 years: 1/100

   In other words: the risk of developing a thrombosis increases tenfold every 20 years of life.

   Female sex is also a risk factor, but not the main one. The likelihood is higher in women than in men, which is attributed to the procoagulant effect of female sex hormones, especially during pregnancy, as well as the use of oral contraceptives in combination with nicotine abuse.

c) **Incorrect.** Virchow's triad is important in the development of thrombosis regardless of the vascular system. Named after its first describer Rudolf Virchow (1821–1902), it is still valid today and describes states of increased thrombosis risk, namely changes in:
   1. Vessel wall
   2. Blood flow
   3. Blood composition

   Changes in one or more of these factors lead to an increased tendency to thrombosis.

d) **Correct.** The Wells score is a measure of the clinical probability of venous thrombosis and is helpful and useful in the initial diagnosis (often in the emergency department) and differential diagnosis of leg swelling of unclear origin. It queries anamnestic risk factors (immobility, previous thrombosis, malignant disease, family history, recent surgery) as well as clinical signs of thrombosis (swelling, difference in circumference, visible venous pattern, tenderness over superficial and deep veins, edema). Each positive finding scores one point; if another differential diagnosis is more likely, two points are subtracted. With a score of two (or more), the clinical probability of thrombosis is high and further diagnostics by sonography are recommended.

e) **Incorrect.** Athletes can also develop thrombosis. Even if none of the usual risk factors (immobility, family history, etc.) are present, there is a venous disease that occurs specifically and especially in athletes. This is called effort thrombosis (thrombosis par effort), another term for Paget-von-Schroetter syndrome. This is a thrombosis in the upper extremity, usually in the context of a thoracic outlet syndrome (TOS). Anatomical causes leading to compression and thus thrombosis include a cervical rib or prominent first rib, as well as malunited clavicle fractures. In addition, training-induced hypertrophy of the pectoralis and scalene muscles can be causative. Thus, sports involving the upper extremity are most commonly affected. Dehydration during intense training or competition can further increase the tendency to thrombosis. The treatment of effort thrombosis is based on the standard strategies for thrombosis, including compression therapy and anticoagulation. Invasive measures are being used more frequently, but overall are still rarely indicated.

Question

3. Which statements about the symptoms and classification of varicosis are correct?

a) Varicose veins may be an aesthetic problem for affected patients, but are usually harmless.
b) Usually, the great saphenous vein (GSV) is affected.
c) Typical complaints range from feelings of tension and swelling, especially in the evening, to dermatitis with skin involvement and itching, or leg ulcers (ulcus cruris).
d) The C-classification is equivalent to the Fontaine classification for PAD, in 4 stages (C1-4).
e) The venous clinical severity score (VCSS) is a classification in which varicosis and CVI are assessed and classified based on clinical signs and symptoms using a point system.

Answers

a) **Correct.** Varicose veins rarely represent a serious medical problem. Nevertheless, patients and their complaints should be taken seriously, and if treatment is desired, insufficient vein segments should be removed early. In addition, as the disease progresses, there may be significant strain and overload of the deep venous system, which can eventually also become insufficient.
b) **Correct.** The GSV is most frequently affected due to its length, usually including one or more tributaries (in the thigh, the anterior and lateral accessory saphenous veins; in the lower leg, the anterior and posterior arcuate veins).

c) **Correct.** This is also often described by the C in the CEAP (Clinical-Etiology-Anatomy-Pathophysiology) classification.
d) **Incorrect.** The classification is equivalent to the Rutherford classification for PAD, in 7 stages (C0–C6), with increasing severity: 0 = asymptomatic, 1 = spider veins, 2 = varicose veins, 3 = edema, 4 = skin changes, 5 = healed ulcer, 6 = active ulcer.
e) **Correct.** In the VCSS, varicosis is assessed according to 10 criteria, with 0–3 points awarded for each feature. Thus, a score of 0–30 can be achieved. The higher the score, the more pronounced the symptoms and findings. Criteria are either based on history (pain, duration of trophic skin lesions, duration and tolerance of compression therapy) or clinical examination (visible varicose veins, edema, induration, inflammation, hyperpigmentation, number and size of ulcers).

Question

4. Which statements about the Hach classification are correct?

a) The Hach classification is a classification of thrombophlebitis.
b) The principle of the Hach classification of trunk varicosis is that it extends from proximal to distal.
c) In the Hach classification of trunk varicosis, all insufficient tributaries are included in the nomenclature.
d) In the Hach classification of trunk varicosis, the length of the insufficient segment is decisive.
e) The Hach classification of trunk varicosis is based solely on morphological criteria.

Answers

a) **Incorrect.** The Hach classification is used to classify trunk varicosis in the legs. There is a classification for the GSV and SSV.
b) **Correct.** The Hach classification of trunk varicosis is based on the extent of the insufficient trunk vein from proximal to distal. This is because varicose vein disease often begins with a saphenofemoral junction insufficiency in the groin (GSV) or popliteal fossa (SSV) and extends distally. Of course, there are also cases where varicose disease originates from insufficient perforating veins along the vein (e.g., in the distal thigh). In such cases, the extent of distal spread is decisive for classification.

c) **Incorrect.** In the Hach classification, accessory veins are included if they are insufficient. Accessory veins include, in the thigh, the anterior (formerly lateral) and posterior (formerly medial) accessory saphenous veins, and in the lower leg, the anterior and posterior distal accessory saphenous veins, formerly called the anterior and posterior arcuate veins. These four accessory veins are routinely included in the Hach classification, typically described as, for example, GSV insufficiency Hach 3 with tributary varicosis (the affected tributary is then specified).

d) **Correct.** In the Hach classification of trunk varicosis, the length of the insufficient segment is decisive. The distal point of insufficiency is considered, assuming the saphenofemoral junction is the starting point. For the great saphenous vein (GSV), the classification is Hach 1–4; for the small saphenous vein (SSV), Hach 1–3.

e) **Correct.** The Hach classification is based on morphological criteria, particularly the length of the insufficient segment and its location. It has proven itself in clinical practice because it is simple and pragmatic and provides guidance for surgical procedures. Functional aspects are not considered. These include, for example:

   I. Type and severity of symptoms
      i. Pain
      ii. Swelling
      iii. Inflammation
      iv. Visible veins
      v. Visible spider veins
      vi. Atrophie blanche
      vii. Livid discoloration
      viii. Ulcers, etc.
   II. Etiology (acquired, congenital)
   III. Perforator insufficiency, tributaries
   IV. Type of outflow disorder
      i. Reflux
      ii. Obstruction
      iii. Aneurysm
      iv. Thrombophlebitis
   V. Initial diagnosis or recurrence

   For a more detailed classification, the CEAP (**c**linical **e**tiology **a**natomy **p**athophysiology) classification has become established. However, this is usually too complex for everyday clinical practice and is primarily used in research and literature.

Question

5. Which statements about perforating veins are correct?

a) There are three perforating veins in the leg that connect the GSV with the deep venous system.
b) The Cockett perforating veins are located in the distal thigh and connect the great saphenous vein to the femoral vein.
c) The Dodd and Boyd (= Sherman) perforating veins connect the great saphenous vein to the deep venous system.
d) The saphenopopliteal junction is not detectable by ultrasound or intraoperatively in about 50% of cases.
e) It is important to document all perforating veins by name before a varicose vein procedure.

Answers

a) **Incorrect.** There are about 150 perforating veins in the leg, of which about 60 are large-caliber and in principle visible by ultrasound. Any perforating vein can be the starting point of trunk varicosis, which is why at least the most important perforating veins in the leg should be named to allow for surgical planning.
b) **Incorrect.** The Cockett perforating veins are located in the lower leg and connect the posterior distal accessory saphenous vein (arcuata posterior) with the posterior tibial veins in the lower leg.
c) **Correct.** The Dodd perforating veins connect the GSV with the femoral vein in the thigh, and the Boyd (= Sherman) perforating veins connect the great saphenous vein with the posterior tibial veins.
d) **Correct.** Studies have shown that the saphenopopliteal junction, compared to the saphenofemoral junction, is not detectable in about 50% of cases. In these cases, the SSV continues proximally as the so-called femoropopliteal vein (also called the "Giacomini vein") and drains from the dorsal thigh medially as a continuation of the posterior accessory saphenous vein into the GSV or directly into the femoral vein. If the SSV does have a junction with the popliteal vein, the femoropopliteal vein is still often present, but much thinner and more superficial.
e) **Incorrect.** Because the venous system shows extraordinary interindividual variability, textbook norms are rare and there are many "normal variants." Therefore, knowing and naming all perforating veins is rarely necessary

and may cause confusion. However, it is important and recommended to mark affected perforating veins preoperatively to facilitate intraoperative identification. When excising the trunk or tributary vein supplied by the perforating vein, selective ligation of the perforator is often unnecessary, so many surgeons do not mark them separately.

Question

6. Which statements about the CEAP classification are correct?

a) The CEAP classification is indispensable in clinical practice for the treatment of varicose veins.
b) In the CEAP classification, clinical subjective complaints of varicose vein disease are taken into account.
c) The location of the affected veins is represented by the A in the CEAP classification.
d) The E in the CEAP classification stands for the number of events (=recurrences).
e) The P in the CEAP classification describes primary varicose veins in more detail.

Answers

a) **Incorrect.** The CEAP classification is a detailed system for classifying venous diseases, primarily of the superficial trunk veins. However, it is mainly used for comparing scientific data and studies; for everyday clinical practice, the classification is too complex in many respects.
b) **Incorrect.** The C in the CEAP classification stands for clinical and describes the severity of the clinical manifestations of venous disease. It ranges from C0 to C6. However, it does not take into account the patient's subjective complaints, but rather records objective findings. For example, C0 means asymptomatic, C2 means visible varicose veins, and C6 means active ulcer.
c) **Correct.** The A refers to the location of the affected veins, divided into superficial (A_s), perforating (A_p), and deep (A_d). In the extended classification, the affected veins are also named (1–5 superficial, 6–16 deep, and 17+18 perforating veins).
d) **Incorrect.** The E stands for Etiology and ranges from congenital (E_c) to primary (E_p) to secondary (E_s). Congenital means present at birth, i.e.,

a venous malformation. Primary varicose veins develop without a trigger; secondary describes varicose veins with a trigger (e.g., previous deep vein thrombosis).

e) **Incorrect.** The P stands for Pathophysiology and is divided into obstruction (P_o), reflux (P_r), and both (P_{or}). Reflux is most commonly mentioned. This is important, among other things, for follow-up or conservative therapy, as compression is the most important measure for reflux, while for obstruction it is used more symptomatically.

Question

7. Which statements about medical compression stockings (MCS) are correct?

a) Compression therapy is an important component of conservative treatment for varicosis.
b) Class II MCS have a compression strength of 40–50 mmHg.
c) For MCS, the abbreviation AD means that the stocking reaches up to the groin.
d) MCS are routinely flat-knitted; for custom-made products, circular-knitted models are prescribed.
e) So-called support stockings are equivalent to class I MCS.

Answers

a) **Correct.** Every varicose vein disease as well as CVI can be treated conservatively. This can be done with medical compression stockings (MCS), or alternatively with elastic compression bandaging.

b) **Incorrect.** Compression classes (CCL) are divided into classes 1–4; the decisive criterion is the compression strength in mmHg:
   I. 19–21 mmHg
   II. up to 32 mmHg
   III. up to 43 mmHg
   IV. > 44 mmHg

   The difference between the perfusion pressure and the compression strength should be at least 50 mmHg, which is why CCL II to IV are contraindicated in many patients with PAD. It is important and noteworthy, however, that the pressure is not the same at every point. The crucial aspect of medical compression stockings is that the pressure decreases from bottom to top, i.e., it is 100% at the ankle, then steadily decreases, and at the thigh only exerts about 40–50% of the compression strength. This is also important for elastic compression bandaging, because if the pressure does not decrease from bottom to top, the bandage can be counterproductive and prevent venous return.

c) **Incorrect.** A to G are defined points on the leg where measurements for stocking fitting are taken. Important in clinical practice for stocking length and prescribing the correct stocking are the following abbreviations:
   - AD: Knee stocking (standard without grip top)
     – ADH: with grip top
   - AG: Thigh or hip stocking (up to just below the groin, standard with approx. 5 cm wide grip top for fixation, hence sometimes also abbreviated as AGH)
     – AGH: with grip top
   - AT: Pantyhose
     – ATU: for pregnancy (U for "Umstand" = maternity)
     – ATM: after delivery (M for "Mutterschutz" = maternity protection)

d) **Incorrect.** Most off-the-shelf products are circular-knitted stockings, which are elastic (long-stretch materials), have a higher resting pressure, and are primarily used for venous diseases. They are knitted in a circular fashion like a sock. Flat-knitted stockings, as the name suggests, are knitted flat, consist of several parts (as with a sweater, for example), and are then sewn together according to the fitting (always custom-made). They are made of stable and less elastic short-stretch materials, have a high working pressure, and are recommended for pronounced edema, especially lipoedema and lymphoedema. Patients with flat-knitted stockings always require a donning aid, as putting on this rather rigid stocking can be very laborious.

e) **Incorrect.** Support stockings are not a medical product and therefore cannot be prescribed. The costs are not covered by health insurance. Support stockings are stockings with light compression intended for people with healthy veins. They are especially recommended in situations of strain, e.g., during long flights or to prevent heavy legs in people with occupational strain (e.g., teachers, surgeons, etc.). They can also be used at home as a substitute for so-called anti-embolism stockings, which are put on partially immobile patients in the hospital. The compression pressure is about 10–15 mmHg, thus lower than that of MCS.

Question

8. Which statements are correct regarding operative varicose vein therapy (stripping)?

a) Sole crossectomy of a trunk varicosis of the GSV Hach IV leads to a high recurrence rate.
b) The "classic" stripping method of the GSV according to Babcock means that the vein is pulled distally by the head screwed onto the probe.
c) The probe is called the Babcock probe.
d) In invaginating stripping, the GSV is extracted proximally.
e) Sole crossectomy without stripping is now obsolete.

Answers

a) **Correct.** Sole crossectomy has a high risk of recurrence; the same applies to crossectomy with stripping of the GSV if a too-long saphenous stump is left. It is therefore recommended to transect the GSV directly in the crossectomy area close to the CFV.
b) **Correct.** In the classic varicose vein operation according to Babcock (first described in 1907), after transecting the GSV and ligating all crossectomy branches, the probe is introduced into the vein from proximal to distal and extracted at the medial malleolus through an additional skin incision. Then, a size-variable knob is screwed onto the probe in the groin, which, when the probe is pulled distally, pulls the vein along with it (called a "carrier"). In the Babcock technique, the entire GSV is generally removed.
c) **Incorrect.** The probe is also called the Nabatoff probe.
d) **Incorrect.** In invaginating stripping, the GSV is also pulled distally; however, no knob is screwed on, but the vein is simply firmly tied to the probe and then extracted. The so-called PIN probe (Perforating Invagination Stripping) according to Oesch is a probe developed specifically for this invaginating technique (1993), which has a loop at the end for fixing the vein and suture. The probe is rigid and, however, did not become established in clinical practice.
e) **Incorrect.** Crossectomy is the basis of operative varicose vein therapy and, in certain indications (e.g., isolated crossectomy insufficiency, i.e., trunk varicosis stage Hach I), is also a sole therapeutic measure. However, in the

long term, a high recurrence rate is to be expected, which is why in most cases an additional procedure such as partial or complete stripping, sclerotherapy, or obliteration is already necessary initially.

Question

9. Which statements about endoluminal laser therapy (ELT) for varicose veins are correct?

a) The use of laser in the endoluminal treatment of varicose veins has been approved in Germany since 1980.
b) The ELVEs®-Painless system is an innovative laser treatment for varicose veins.
c) Endoluminal laser therapy generates significantly higher temperatures than radiofrequency ablation.
d) Laser therapy is particularly suitable for insufficiencies of the GSV in stage Hach IV.
e) The probe tip should be placed below the junction of the superficial epigastric vein.

Answers

a) **Incorrect.** ELT has been approved in Germany since 1999 and has been increasingly used since then. The principle is the application of heat intraluminally to achieve obliteration and adhesion of the vein wall. Temperatures of up to 700 degrees Celsius are generated at the catheter tip.
b) **Correct.** The ELVEs® system from the German laser manufacturer biolitec AG is a further development of the conventional laser system. The abbreviation stands for **E**ndo **L**aser **Ve**in **S**ystem. The special feature of this system is that, according to the manufacturer, the probe delivers the energy specifically to the vein wall and, due to a lower penetration depth, causes fewer skin burns.
c) **Correct.** Laser therapy generates temperatures of up to 700 degrees Celsius, while radiofrequency ablation generates temperatures up to 120 degrees. This could be a reason for the slightly higher number of skin burns after laser therapy (1–4.8%) compared to radiofrequency ablation (0–0.36%).
d) **Incorrect.** Endoluminal procedures are particularly suitable for the GSV at the thigh up to just below the knee joint. As soon as the vein is more superficial, there is a significantly higher complication rate with skin burns

and discolorations, so both laser and radiofrequency therapy are only recommended up to just below the knee joint. For this reason, the GSV is usually punctured just below the knee joint, the probe is then advanced to just below the crossectomy junction, and the endoluminal therapy is performed under controlled withdrawal of the probe.

e) **Correct.** In endoluminal procedures, the probe tip should be placed about 1 cm below the crossectomy junction. The superficial epigastric vein serves as a landmark, as it is the uppermost crossectomy branch and is clearly visible running mediocranially.

Question

10. Which statements about endovenous radiofrequency ablation (RFA) are correct?

a) RFA is preferably used to treat the small saphenous vein (SSV).
b) The most commonly used device is the VNUS ClosureFAST™.
c) Due to the significantly lower heat generation compared to laser therapy, infiltration of a tumescent solution is not necessary.
d) Recurrence rates after RFA treatment are significantly lower than after conventional stripping surgery.
e) In so-called bipolar RFA by Celon/Olympus, fewer burns occur than with segmental RFA by Medtronic.

Answers

a) **Incorrect.** In endoluminal procedures (available since 1998), including RFA, the GSV at the thigh up to just below the knee joint is preferably treated. The superficially located GSV at the lower leg should, if possible, not be treated with endoluminal procedures. The reason is that RFA generates pronounced heat, and if the vein is superficial, the risk of skin burns is very high.

b) **Correct.** The VNUS ClosureFAST™ from Medtronic is the most commonly used device in Germany. Through the repeatedly applicable and controlled heat development of 90–120 degrees Celsius, the collagen of the vein wall contracts and the vein closes.

c) **Incorrect.** Tumescent solution is also used in RFA, especially for pain management. But also for compression of the vein and thus improved efficacy of the endoluminal therapy as well as for skin protection, the solution should be infiltrated. Even with RFA, due to heat development of up to 120 degrees Celsius, skin burns are quite possible.

d) **Incorrect.** Long-term results regarding recurrence rates after RFA, especially compared to conventional crossectomy and stripping, rather indicate a higher recurrence rate after RFA. These range between 2–20%, whereas after technically flawless crossectomy, a recurrence rate of less than 5% after 10 years is reported. However, technical advances, especially in RFA but also in EVLA, suggest that further long-term results with lower recurrence rates will be published in the future.
e) **Incorrect.** In bipolar RFA, an alternating current flows at the probe tip located in the vein. The probe can also measure resistance changes in the vein wall, so the device switches off automatically at a certain resistance. The purpose is to reduce side effects outside the varicose vein to be treated, especially skin discolorations and burns. However, there is no clear evidence that this procedure has fewer skin complications than segmental RFA by Medtronic (VNUS ClosureFAST™). In segmental ablation, a 7 cm long segment at the probe tip is heated by radiofrequency energy, and the catheter is gradually withdrawn from proximal to distal.

Question

11. Which statements about sclerotherapy of varicose veins are correct?

a) Polidocanol (Aethoxysklerol®) is the most commonly used liquid sclerosing agent for so-called spider vein varicosis in Germany.
b) Contraindications for sclerotherapy include advanced PAD, diabetes mellitus, or known allergies.
c) Sclerotherapy is free of side effects and can be used without reservation.
d) Polidocanol is also used in foam sclerotherapy, here in foamed form.
e) The ClariVein® method is a combination of mechanical and chemical varicose vein treatment.

Answers

a) **Correct.** Polidocanol (Aethoxysklerol®) is the only sclerosing agent approved in Germany and is available in concentrations of 0.25%, 0.5%, 1%, and 3%.
b) **Correct.** Advanced PAD in stage 3 or 4, diabetes mellitus with diabetic micro- and macroangiopathy, and known allergy to Aethoxysklerol® are the

most common contraindications. It should also not be used in cases of multiple drug allergies.

c) **Incorrect.** Sclerotherapy also has risks, especially skin reactions such as hyperpigmentation, redness, or allergic reactions. Discolorations due to polidocanol and, in extreme cases, necrosis can also occur, which must be mentioned during the informed consent discussion. This is particularly important when the indication is for cosmetic reasons, which is the majority of cases.
The risk of hyperpigmentation and skin effects is reported in the literature as up to 80%, but most skin changes disappear after 1 year. Only about 1–5% result in permanent cutaneous reactions.
d) **Correct.** In foam sclerotherapy, polidocanol is foamed using the so-called double-syringe technique (DSS according to Tessari). The ratio of air to liquid is usually 4:1. The larger the vessel to be sclerosed, the higher the concentration of polidocanol should be (available from 0.25% to 3%).
e) **Correct.** This is also called mechano-chemical ablation, a combination of endoluminal and sclerosing procedures. The principle of this approach is that the inner vein wall is irritated with a catheter, at the tip of which is a rotating wire, and then sclerosed with foam. The system of catheter, wire, and application device is called the ClariVein® system by the manufacturer MeritMedical. The advantage is that no heat is generated and therefore no tumescent solution needs to be used.

Question

12. Which statements about thrombophlebitis are correct?

a) Thrombophlebitis of the GSV must be treated with therapeutic anticoagulation and compression therapy for at least 3 months, regardless of its extent.
b) So-called thrombophlebitis saltans (migrans) is a harmless disease and often occurs after multiple venipunctures.
c) Mondor's phlebitis is a thrombophlebitis of the superficial epigastric or thoracoepigastric vein.
d) Fondaparinux (Arixtra®) may be indicated postoperatively as anticoagulation after crossectomy of the GSV with involvement of the deep venous system for three months.
e) As soon as thrombophlebitis of the GSV reaches the crossectomy or extends into the deep venous system, emergency crossectomy is indicated.

Answers

a) **Incorrect.** Uncomplicated thrombophlebitis of the GSV generally does not require anticoagulation. Only if it is longer than > 5 cm is prophylactic anticoagulation with fondaparinux (Arixtra®) 2.5 mg once daily for 4–6 weeks recommended in addition to the basically indicated compression therapy. However, if the thrombophlebitis is < 3 cm from the crossectomy, therapeutic anticoagulation for 3 months is indicated.

b) **Incorrect.** Thrombophlebitis saltans (also called phlebitis migrans) is a serious disease in which recurrent thrombophlebitides of the leg and especially the arm veins occur. They typically occur spontaneously, heal within a short time without sequelae, only to reappear elsewhere. Especially in young patients, mainly men, a malignant underlying disease (e.g., testicular tumor) must be considered. Other typical malignancies regularly associated with thrombophlebitis migrans are bronchial and pancreatic carcinoma as well as leukemia.

c) **Correct.** Mondor's phlebitis is a thrombophlebitis in the thoracic area, the cause of which is not fully understood. Most commonly affected are the superficial epigastric or thoracoepigastric veins. Clinically, this manifests as hardening and redness along the course of the named veins. Possible causes include breast surgery, breast cancer, or thrombophilias (anticardiolipin antibody syndrome, protein C deficiency). Therapy, in addition to searching for the cause and further diagnostics, is usually symptomatic; anticoagulation or invasive measures are only indicated in exceptional cases.

d) **Correct.** Regarding postoperative management after crossectomy of the GSV with involvement of the deep venous system, many surgeons and authors recommend postoperative management as for deep vein thrombosis. This means therapeutic anticoagulation for at least three months. For this, in addition to low-molecular-weight heparin, Arixtra® in therapeutic dosage (7.5 mg once daily) or a NOAC or phenprocoumon can be prescribed. In principle, it can be argued that after crossectomy, no further anticoagulation is necessary, as the risk of embolization should be reduced or eliminated by the crossectomy. Arguments for therapeutic anticoagulation for three months, however, are that the GSV, which is usually left in situ, still has further connections to the deep venous system along its course, and the risk of further embolizations exists via these.

e) **Incorrect.** Opinions differ regarding the necessity of urgent or emergency crossectomy in thrombophlebitis with crossectomy involvement. Some advocate a generous indication for surgery as soon as the thrombus reaches or extends beyond the crossectomy. Others favor conservative therapy and consider it sufficient if the indication is made early and the measures are carried out adequately. Therapy includes therapeutic anticoagulation, for example with a NOAC or Arixtra® 7.5 mg once daily.

Question

13. Which statements about May-Thurner syndrome are correct?

a) May-Thurner syndrome is a malignant disease of the vein wall.
b) May-Thurner syndrome occurs preferentially in young men on the right side.
c) The causative pelvic vein spur can be well visualized preoperatively by CT angiography.
d) After successful thrombolysis or thrombectomy, a stent should definitely be implanted to eliminate the pelvic vein spur.
e) The Wallstent® is most often chosen for treatment of the pelvic vein spur.

Answers

a) **False.** May-Thurner syndrome refers to a descending form of pelvic vein thrombosis caused by a so-called pelvic vein spur. Robert May (1912–1984) was an Austrian surgeon, and Josef Thurner (1927), also from Innsbruck, was a pathologist. Incidentally, the names are pronounced in German, not, as is often observed, in English. The syndrome named after them was described in 1957. However, Rudolf Virchow had already described in 1851 that left-sided pelvic vein thrombosis occurs significantly more frequently than right-sided.
b) **False.** May-Thurner syndrome preferentially occurs on the left side in young women. The cause of the left-sided descending pelvic vein thrombosis (= May-Thurner syndrome) is the so-called "pelvic vein spur," which arises from the crossing of the left common iliac vein beneath the right common iliac artery. These are scarred changes of the pelvic vein at the crossing point, caused by continuous compression due to arterial pulsations.
c) **False.** The causative pelvic vein spur can at best be visualized intraoperatively after successful thrombectomy of the pelvic vein using phlebography. Preoperatively, visualization is generally not possible, as the spur cannot be delineated due to the thrombotic material.
d) **False.** In principle, it is possible to implant a stent. Due to the good patency rates, some authors recommend always placing a stent, even if, after successful recanalization, the stenosis appears only mild. Others argue that the

stent is a foreign body and should only be used in most young women if the stenosis caused by the pelvic vein spur is of a higher degree.

e) **Correct.** The Wallstent® from Boston Scientific Corporate is a self-expanding stent made of the precious metal alloy Elgiloy® (non-magnetic, cobalt-chromium-nickel-molybdenum). This stent is very robust, has high radial or tensile strength, and is preferably used in central veins, in the supraaortic and iliac arteries, in the biliary system, and tracheobronchially. It is available in lengths from 23–145 mm and diameters from 5–24 mm. In the venous system, it should, if possible, be "overdilated" by about 10% to keep the restenosis rate as low as possible. The Wallstent® was originally developed for the gastrointestinal tract (esophagus), bile ducts, and bronchial system due to its high radial strength. For venous indications, especially May-Thurner syndrome, stents specifically developed for the venous system are now available, e.g., Venovo™/Bard; VICI Venous®/Boston Scientific; Sinus XL®/Optimed; Zilver® Vena™/Cook Medical; BeYond Venous®/Bentley.

Question

14. Which statements about the relationship between PAD and venous diseases are correct?

a) The manifestation of pelvic-leg type PAD is a risk factor for the development of deep vein thrombosis of the leg.
b) Elevated cholesterol levels are a risk factor for both PAD and DVT.
c) Diabetics have an increased risk of developing PAD compared to the general population, but not of suffering a DVT.
d) With every examination for suspected DVT, an orienting examination of the arteries should also be performed.
e) Thrombophlebitis in young smokers can be the first indication of the presence of thromboangiitis obliterans (TAO).

Answers

a) **Correct.** PAD, and especially the number of affected vascular regions, is a risk factor for the development and progression of deep vein thrombosis of the leg. In the general population, the incidence of deep vein thrombosis of the leg is estimated at about 0.1%/year; in PAD with one affected vascular region, it is about 0.3%, with two affected regions already 1–2%, and with three regions about 3–5%. A possible explanation is the reduction in mobility that accompanies increasing severity of PAD. However, it could also be a bias, namely that the severity of PAD is not the decisive influencing factor, but rather the generally higher age of the affected patients. In other words: as is well known, age is the greatest risk factor for the development of DVT and also for the severity and number of affected vascular regions in PAD.

b) **False.** Elevated cholesterol and lipid levels are a risk factor for the development of PAD, but not for DVT. Besides age as a non-modifiable risk factor, overweight and smoking are the most important and at the same time modifiable risk factors for the development of both PAD and DVT.
c) **Correct.** Diabetes mellitus is not a risk factor for the development of DVT.
d) **Correct.** The symptoms that may lead to the suspicion of DVT (pain, sensory disturbances, skin discoloration, movement disorders) can also be caused by PAD or an arterial occlusion. Therefore, the pulse status and arterial flow signals at the foot should always be assessed. If abnormalities are found, further investigations should follow.
e) **Correct.** TAO, as a very rare special form of PAD in young (mostly male) smokers, can present with recurrent thrombophlebitis as the first clinical sign. These phlebitides, also known as thrombophlebitis saltans, can also occur paraneoplastically, e.g., in testicular tumors in the same patient group.

Question

15. Which statements about the classification of deep vein thrombosis are correct?

a) The most common form of DVT in the lower extremity is ascending thrombosis.
b) The classification of ascending DVT is into 4 levels.
c) May-Thurner syndrome typically leads to a descending thrombosis.
d) In thoracic outlet syndrome (TOS), a descending thrombosis can also occur.
e) In trans-fascial thrombosis, there is, in addition to DVT, secondary involvement of the superficial veins.

Answers

a) **Correct.** In ascending DVT, as the name suggests, the thrombosis ascends. It usually originates in the lower leg and migrates upward, essentially as a propagation thrombosis due to gravity and stasis. In the upper extremity, ascending and descending thromboses occur in roughly equal proportions.

However, upper extremity thromboses account for only about 1–4% of all thromboses.

b) **Correct.** The classification of ascending DVT is typically from distal to proximal in levels 1–4:
   I. Lower leg
   II. up to the knee
   III. up to the thigh (but below the groin)
   IV. up to the groin (and beyond)
c) **Correct.** In May-Thurner syndrome, a descending thrombosis typically occurs, originating from a pelvic vein spur. This is most often on the left side, at the crossing of the left vein with the right common iliac artery. This typically results in an obstruction at this site, which promotes thrombosis formation. Compared to ascending thrombosis, this form extends from proximal to distal.
d) **Correct.** In TOS with venous involvement, a descending thrombosis regularly occurs, caused by stenosis at the upper thoracic aperture. In "Paget-von-Schrötter syndrome," a descending thrombosis also typically occurs, as here too there is usually an anatomical or functional obstruction.
e) **False.** In trans-fascial thrombosis, a thrombosis of a superficial vein (= thrombophlebitis) leads via the perforating veins to a thrombosis of the deep venous system. This form of thrombosis is much rarer than the ascending type, but about as common as the descending variant.

Question

16. Which statements about the conservative therapy of DVT are correct?

a) In duplex sonographic follow-up 6 months after initial diagnosis of a 4-level vein thrombosis, more than 50% of patients show at least partial recanalization
b) Extending oral anticoagulation beyond 6 months usually offers no benefit for the patient in uncomplicated 4-level vein thrombosis.
c) Eliquis® (apixaban) is approved for deep vein thrombosis at a permanent dose of 10 mg twice daily for 6 months.
d) Compression therapy for DVT should be discontinued at the same time as anticoagulation.
e) With anticoagulation using phenprocoumon (Marcumar®), weight-adjusted administration of a low-molecular-weight heparin (LMWH) should be given until the therapeutic range is reached (Quick 20–30%, INR 2–3).

Answers

a) **False.** About 50% of patients with ascending deep vein thrombosis of the leg still show occlusive processes and valve damage of the deep veins in duplex sonographic follow-up after 6 months. This was shown in the CaVenT study. Nevertheless, about 30–40% of patients experience partial or complete recanalization of the thrombosed veins, so the importance of conservative therapy with consistent compression therapy and anticoagulation should be explained and made clear to the patient. Not every patient benefits from an intravenous procedure such as thrombectomy or lysis therapy, especially considering the sometimes considerable risk of complications.

b) **Correct.** In uncomplicated deep vein thrombosis of the leg without special risk factors, guidelines recommend discontinuing anticoagulation after 6 months. The recurrence risk is statistically less than 3%/year. If risk factors are present (recurrent thrombosis, persistently elevated D-dimers, known thrombophilia such as antiphospholipid syndrome or factor V Leiden syndrome or prothrombin mutation), the recurrence risk is estimated at more than 3%/year and the recommendation to continue anticoagulation therapy is made more generously. Ultimately, however, there are no strict rules; an individual decision should be made.

c) **False.** Eliquis® (apixaban) is administered for deep vein thrombosis for the first 7 days at a dose of 2 × 10 mg, then for 3–6 months at a dose of 5 mg twice daily.

d) **False.** In contrast to anticoagulation, which according to guidelines is recommended for 3–6 months (in exceptional cases longer) depending on the extent, symptoms, and genesis of DVT, compression therapy should be continued for a longer period. According to current studies, this leads to a significant reduction in the risk of post-thrombotic syndrome (PTS).

e) **Correct.** In contrast to the new oral anticoagulants (NOACs), where overlapping heparinization is not necessary, this is urgently indicated with oral anticoagulation using phenprocoumon. The reason is the procoagulant effect of phenprocoumon in the first hours to few days. This is because Marcumar® inhibits not only the vitamin K-dependent synthesis of coagulation factors (factors II, VII, IX, and X) but also that of protein C and S. The latter are anticoagulant and have a much shorter half-life (5–10 h) than the coagulation factors (2–3 days). Therefore, coagulation activation occurs in the first days, making heparinization necessary. In addition to the risk of thrombosis, the risk of developing "Marcumar necrosis" also increases. This is a very rare but quite serious development of skin and tissue necrosis.

Question

17. Which statements about Paget-von-Schrötter syndrome are correct?

a) Paget-von-Schrötter syndrome is an acute thrombosis of the arm veins.
b) Paget-von-Schrötter syndrome occurs especially in young athletes.
c) The arm veins are usually free of thrombus in Paget-von-Schrötter syndrome.
d) Paget-von-Schrötter syndrome is also internationally referred to as thoracic inlet syndrome.
e) Paget-von-Schrötter syndrome usually occurs on the left.

Answers

a) **Correct.** Paget-von-Schrötter syndrome describes an acute thrombosis of the veins in the shoulder and arm area, which manifests as swelling of the arm and pain in the shoulder and upper arm.
b) **Correct.** Paget-von-Schrötter syndrome is often described in young, athletic, and muscular men. Another term is "thrombosis par effort," which expresses the acute exertion and strain as the cause.
c) **Correct.** In contrast to venous thromboses of the lower extremity, where more than 90% are ascending thromboses and the distal veins are involved, thrombosis of the upper extremity veins usually arises in the subclavian or axillary vein, with the veins below generally free of thrombus.
d) **False.** The previously common term "thoracic inlet syndrome" is no longer used today. The term TOS (thoracic outlet syndrome) is now common, with distinction into venous, arterial, and neurogenic TOS. Instead of the previously common term thoracic inlet syndrome, the term venous TOS is now used.
e) **False.** Paget-von-Schrötter syndrome most commonly affects the dominant side, i.e., the right. This is further evidence for the mechanical cause or compression-related etiology in the primarily loaded and more muscular extremity.

Question

18. Which statements about phlegmasia coerulea dolens (PCD) are correct?

a) Phlegmasia coerulea dolens (PCD) is a venous emergency.
b) Phlegmasia coerulea dolens (PCD) typically occurs in young women.

c) In about 1% of deep vein thromboses of the leg, phlegmasia coerulea dolens (PCD) develops.
d) In phlegmasia coerulea dolens (PCD), fasciotomy is more important than venous recanalization.
e) Patients with recurrent thromboses are particularly at risk of developing phlegmasia coerulea dolens (PCD).

Answers

a) **Correct.** In phlegmasia coerulea dolens (PCD), a thrombotic occlusion of the deep veins of a limb, usually the lower limb, leads to complete interruption of venous outflow. Due to the increase in tissue swelling beyond systolic blood pressure, arterial perfusion disturbance develops in the course of PCD. Emergency surgery is then indicated to save the limb. The decisive factor for the urgency of treatment is therefore not the thrombosis itself, but the increase in swelling and ultimately the restriction or cessation of arterial perfusion.
b) **False.** Phlegmasia coerulea dolens (PCD) does occur in young women, but is not concentrated in this patient group. In fact, patients of any age can be affected; men are even somewhat more frequently affected.
c) **False.** Phlegmasia coerulea dolens (PCD) is much rarer, but is also not infrequently misdiagnosed. The typical clinical presentation of massive leg swelling with (beginning) bluish discoloration is not proof of phlegmasia coerulea dolens (PCD), but occurs in the early stage of a large proportion of venous thromboses. The decisive criterion for phlegmasia coerulea dolens (PCD) is the pulse status: palpable foot pulses or an ankle-brachial index (ABI) > 0.9 are exclusion criteria for PCD. Nevertheless, compression, elevation, and strict close monitoring of the limb are essential, but by definition this is not phlegmasia coerulea dolens (PCD). In manifest PCD, conservative therapy is contraindicated and is associated with a mortality of almost 50% and a risk of limb loss of > 80%.
d) **False.** There are colleagues who always perform fasciotomy in phlegmasia coerulea dolens (PCD). Others argue, however, that after recanalization of the venous pathway, swelling subsides within minutes and fasciotomy can be omitted. Nevertheless, it must be considered that, depending on the duration of ischemia, a more or less pronounced reperfusion syndrome can develop, so opening the compartments is recommended in many cases. At the very least, no one can be blamed, even in the case of prophylactic fasciotomy; the situation is different in the event of limb loss due to failure

to perform fasciotomy. Surgical venous recanalization is still considered the gold standard despite increasingly available interventional methods, as thrombosis can be eliminated most quickly this way. The key is successful recanalization of the pelvic segment with outflow from the profunda territory; the femoropopliteal pathway should also be thrombectomized, but does not necessarily have to be patent if unsuccessful.

e) **False.** Patients particularly at risk are those with malignant diseases; more than a third of patients suffer from a curatively or often palliatively treated tumor disease. Previously undiagnosed malignancies, especially from the visceral surgical and gynecological fields, are also not uncommon, so PCD should prompt a search for tumors. Other risk factors are congenital and acquired thrombophilias. Recurrent thrombosis itself is not a risk factor on its own.

Question

19. Which statements about venous leg ulcer (UCV) are correct?

a) Venous leg ulcer (UCV) is, after arterial ulcer, the most common type of ulcer on the lower leg.
b) Venous leg ulcer (UCV) is usually located on the lateral lower leg.
c) Compared to PAD, venous leg ulcer (UCV) is not a disease that occurs more frequently with age.
d) Venous leg ulcer (UCV) is classified according to Widmer.
e) The ESCHAR study showed that E. coli is the most common pathogen in venous leg ulcer (UCV).

Answers

a) **False.** UCV is the most common form of ulcer and accounts for > 50% of all chronic wounds on the lower leg. The arterially induced form (ulcus cruris arteriosum, UCA) as well as the mixed form of both (ulcus cruris mixtum, UCM) are significantly less common. Other causes such as infections, inflammations, trauma, or malignant diseases are exceptions in the pathogenesis of leg ulcers.

b) **False.** Compared to the purely arterial form, UCV is mainly located medially, but can also occur laterally or circumferentially. The latter is known as a gaiter ulcer. The predominantly medial localization is due to the pathogenesis and development in the context of chronic venous insufficiency

(CVI), where the GSV is the main affected and insufficient vein running medially and originating in the area of the medial malleolus.

c) **False.** The likelihood of developing a venous leg ulcer also shows an age dependency. This was demonstrated by the results of the Bonn Vein Study. According to this, the prevalence
   I. in the general population was about 0.5%,
   II. in those < 40 years old was < 0.1%, and
   III. in those > 80 years old was 4–5%.

   Possible reasons for this age dependency include, among others, the increased risk with age of suffering a thrombosis of the deep or superficial venous system, developing varicosis or thrombophlebitis, as well as generally poorer and delayed wound healing.
d) **False.** The Widmer classification is a staging system for chronic venous insufficiency (CVI) and is divided into I–III. In stage I, there are no skin affections yet (edema, corona phlebectatica = visibly ectatic veins at the foot margin, stasis eczema, dermatoliposclerosis), and stage III refers to UCV. IIIa describes the healed and IIIb the active ulcer. Stage IIIa according to Widmer corresponds to stage C5 of the CEAP classification, stage IIIb = C6 according to CEAP.
e) **False.** The ESCHAR study (Comparison of surgery and compression with compression alone in chronic venous ulceration) was an RCT in which healing of UCV under compression therapy alone and with additional removal of varicose veins was investigated. Significantly better ulcer healing was demonstrated in the "Surgery" group both after 1 and after 4 years. This has led to a certain rethinking and more proactive approach among treating physicians (primarily vascular surgeons and dermatologists). Since then, the indication for invasive varicose vein therapy in UCV is made early and generously.

Question

20. Which statements about ongoing studies on venous diseases are correct?

a) The CARAVAGGIO study compares apixaban with dalteparin in the treatment of thrombosis in cancer patients.
b) The MUFFIN-PTS study investigates the influence of a carbohydrate-rich diet on the course of CVI.
c) The VEINS study investigates which influencing factors exist for the development of venous leg ulcers (UCV) in chronic venous insufficiency (CVI).

d) The VenUS-6 study compares different compression techniques in UCV.
e) The CASS study compares stripping of the GSV with compression therapy.

Answers

a) **Correct.** In the CARAVAGGIO study, patients with venous thrombosis and underlying malignancy are randomized and double-blinded for 6 months to receive either apixaban (Eliquis®, day 1–7 2×10 mg, from day 8 2×5 mg) or dalteparin (Fragmin®, 150 IU/kg). The primary endpoint was regression of thrombosis or recurrence rate. Bleeding complications were also compared, with apixaban being non-inferior in all endpoints. There was also a trend toward a lower risk of recurrent thrombosis with apixaban, although this was not significant. Long-term results of the study are still pending.
b) **False.** The MUFFIN-PTS study (Micronized Purified Flavonoid Fraction for the Treatment of Post-Thrombotic) investigates the influence of flavonoids compared to placebo medication on the course and development of CVI after venous thrombosis. Flavonoids are plant substances that have been observed to have a venotonic (= stabilizing) effect. It has also been reported that flavonoids may be more effective than compression therapy, especially in chronic congestion symptoms. This would be of considerable importance in patients with arterial and venous (so-called "mixed") congestion problems, as compression therapy should not or only cautiously be performed in this selected patient group.
c) **Correct.** The VEINS study (venous insufficiency in South Florida) is a cohort study in Florida, in which patients with CVI are included and followed for > 5 years. The aim is to determine which factors and patient characteristics influence the development of UCV, in order to take appropriate prophylactic measures in the future. Especially in view of the increasing incidence of UCV and the rising costs and consumption of resources (material, personnel, inpatient capacities) for chronic wounds, there is great interest in providing relief and acting prophylactically.
d) **Correct.** The VenUS-6 study is a multicenter randomized study in which patients with UCV are included and treated with different compression methods. It is a three-arm study; compression is performed either with compression bandages, medical compression stockings/tights of class II or III. The probability and speed of healing are the main focus of this study.
e) **False.** In the CASS study (CyanoAcrylate closure versus Surgical Stripping for incompetent saphenous veins), endoluminal therapy with cyanoacrylate adhesive using the VenaSeal™ closure system (Medtronic) and stripping

of the GSV are compared. It is a multicenter randomized study, with the primary endpoint being the recurrence rate after 3 months. Secondary endpoints are recurrence-free survival after > 2 years, as well as satisfaction, wound infections, etc.

Question

21. Which statements about the evidence comparing surgical versus endoluminal treatment methods for varicosis are correct?

a) Randomized studies have shown that the rate of saphenofemoral recurrence after open surgery (crossectomy with stripping of the GSV (C&S)) was higher than after endovenous procedures (RFA and EVLA).
b) According to current studies, the duration of incapacity for work after ELV appears to be shorter than after C&S.
c) The VenaSeal™ closure procedure is the only non-thermal endovenous method that also shows good results with GSV diameters > 6 mm in the saphenofemoral region.
d) According to current evidence, no compression therapy is necessary after RFA or EVLA compared to C&S.
e) The SF-36 questionnaire is frequently used in comparative studies on the treatment of varicosis.

Answers

a) **False.** Several randomized studies have compared crossectomy with stripping (C&S) and endoluminal procedures (ELV) (RFA and EVLA). Some studies showed a higher recurrence rate after endovenous therapy (e.g., Flessenkämper et al., 2013: after 6 months: ELV 31.5% vs. C&S 1.6%; Rass et al., 2012: after 2 years: EVLA 17.8% vs. C&S 1.3%). Other studies showed no significant differences. It is noteworthy that none of the available studies reported a higher recurrence rate after C&S, which strongly suggests that, regarding saphenofemoral recurrence, there is a certain advantage of surgical procedures over endoluminal applications.
b) **Correct.** The duration of postoperative incapacity for work is shorter after ELV than after C&S. This may be due to smaller access routes, fewer hematomas and wound infections, and the avoidance of general anesthesia. However, some authors suspect a bias due to more complicated and complex cases being treated under inpatient conditions with C&S. On the other

hand, uncomplicated cases are primarily treated on an outpatient basis in private practice using endovenous procedures.

c) **False.** In the VenaSeal™ closure procedure, n-butyl cyanoacrylate is used as a non-sclerosing agent and injected into the varicose vein. Studies have shown comparable results with this procedure to thermal methods and the injection of sclerosing agents (polidocanol). However, it is currently not approved for varicose veins with diameters > 6 mm.

d) **False.** Compression therapy is recommended after both surgical and endovascular treatment of varicosis. According to current studies, this leads to a significant reduction in postoperative or post-interventional edema, pain, and a shorter duration of incapacity for work. There is consensus regarding the compression strength used; medical compression stockings of class II are recommended. However, there are no clear guidelines regarding the duration of compression therapy. In Germany, it is often recommended for 2–4 weeks, while in Anglo-American countries usually only for about 7 days. However, current data suggest that one week is too short after both stripping and endovenous procedures. The only exception appears to be the non-thermal, non-sclerosing treatment with the VenaSeal™ closure procedure and n-butyl cyanoacrylate, where a compression duration of more than 7 days does not provide any relevant advantages.
It is also worth mentioning here that eccentric compression using foam and pads applied along the course of the treated varicose vein offers advantages over compression therapy alone and should be offered.

e) **Correct.** The SF-36 questionnaire is the most frequently used questionnaire in science to assess and compare patient well-being. It is also often referred to as a score for determining patient-related outcomes (PRO). It consists of 36 questions covering 8 areas, including psychological, social, and physical well-being, pain, general health perception, etc. The score ranges from 0–100, with 100 indicating no health limitations and 0 the worst health status. Another important and frequently used score in science is the EuroQol-5D score, which assesses and rates 5 areas: mobility, self-care, daily activities, physical pain, and psychological problems.

Acute Limb Ischemia (ALI) 9

1. Which statements about the epidemiology of acute limb ischemia (ALI) are correct?

a) The incidence of ALI is approximately 10/100,000 inhabitants per year.
b) About 5% of patients with ALI lose the limb as a result.
c) The majority of ALI cases are due to arterial thrombosis in pre-existing atherosclerosis.
d) The lower extremity is the most common site of embolic occlusion, accounting for > 50%.
e) A COVID-19 infection increases the risk of limb loss in ALI.

Answers

a) **Correct.** In industrialized countries, ALI has an annual incidence of about 10/100,000 inhabitants and accounts for approximately 10–15% of inpatient cases in vascular surgery departments. The average age was about 50 years in the 1950s and has steadily increased in recent years. It is currently around 70 years.
b) **Incorrect.** The risk of limb loss is 10–40%. ALI caused by embolism in particular carries a high risk of amputation. This is due to the usually pronounced ischemic symptoms (complete ischemia), which in turn are attributable to a lack of collateralization.
c) **Incorrect.** The most common cause of ALI is arterial embolism (80–90%), while arterial thrombosis is much less common at 10–20%. Embolism is most often of cardiac origin, i.e., arrhythmias or valvular disease. Therefore, the diagnostic workup for embolic vascular occlusion includes

S. Regus, *Vascular Surgery: Questions and Answers*,
https://doi.org/10.1007/978-3-662-73387-5_9

performing an ECG (usually a long-term ECG) and an echocardiogram to search for the embolic source. Other possible embolic sources include aortoiliac or popliteal aneurysms, which are less common than cardiac causes but should be ruled out. This is especially important if cardiac causes have been excluded. To rule out upstream aneurysms, CT angiography is recommended, as it is usually the fastest available and most reliable. Aortic dissections, which can also lead to ALI, can also be visualized—especially if the iliac-femoral axis is involved or if there is occlusion or collapse of the true lumen. Malignant emboli, such as from an atrial myxoma, are extremely rare. Some surgeons therefore routinely request histological examination of emboli or thrombi removed intraoperatively.

d) **Incorrect.** The distribution of embolic occlusion sites is as follows:
   1. Most commonly, about 60% affect the extra- and intracranial vessels of the head,
   2. followed by the lower extremities at about 20%,
   3. the remaining 20% of embolic events affect the upper extremity and visceral vessels.

   The fact that the supra-aortic branches are most commonly affected is probably due to their anatomical location and the fact that they are the first branches of the aortic arch. The very rare involvement of visceral vessels can also be explained anatomically. However, why the upper extremities, as supra-aortic branches, are much less frequently affected than the cerebral vessels cannot be explained anatomically.

e) **Incorrect.** According to current studies, the combined primary endpoint (30-day mortality and amputation rate) is significantly higher in patients with a COVID infection, but this is due to the high mortality and not the amputation rate. The risk of limb loss or death within 30 days of diagnosis in ALI with concomitant COVID infection is about 50–60%, compared to 20–25% without COVID infection. However, the risk of limb loss, regardless of infection status, is about 15%.

2. Which statements about the classification of acute limb ischemia are correct?

a) Acute ischemia is classified according to Rutherford into stages I–III.
b) The TASC (**T**ran**s**atlantic Inter**s**ociety **C**onsensus) classification uses stages 0–6.
c) Acute ischemia is defined as acute symptoms lasting < 4 weeks.

d) In Rutherford I ischemia, revascularization should be performed within 48 hours at the latest.
e) In Rutherford III ischemia, revascularization should be performed quickly, within one hour, otherwise the limb is at risk.

Answers

a) **Correct.** The classification is based on clinical findings, especially sensitivity and motor function, as well as the presence of arterial and venous Doppler signals. In stage I, sensitivity and motor function are fully preserved, and both arterial and venous signals can be detected with a pencil probe. In stage III, sensitivity and motor function are completely lost, and neither arterial nor venous signals are detectable. Stage II is subdivided into IIa and IIb, with only sensitivity impaired in IIa, and both sensitivity and motor function impaired in IIb.
b) **Incorrect.** The TASC classification corresponds to the Rutherford classification and also uses stages I–III.
c) **Incorrect.** Acute ischemia is defined as clinical symptoms lasting less than 14 days; if symptoms persist longer, it is considered a chronic circulatory disorder. Chronic ischemia is then classified according to Rutherford stages 0–6 or Fontaine stages I–IV.
d) **Incorrect.** Rutherford I ischemia represents a compensated circulatory situation that does not require urgent intervention. Symptoms occur only with exertion; patients are usually asymptomatic at rest. If symptoms persist for more than 14 days, from day 15 onward it is considered a chronic circulatory disorder according to Fontaine stage II or Rutherford I–III (depending on the degree of walking distance limitation).
e) **Incorrect.** Rutherford III ischemia is an irreversible circulatory disorder, so urgent amputation is indicated. Surgical or endovascular revascularization procedures are contraindicated in advanced and irreversible tissue damage, as subsequent systemic reperfusion syndrome can endanger the patient's life and mortality is extremely high.

3. Which statements about the etiology of acute limb ischemia are correct?

a) The causes of arterial occlusion include embolism or thrombosis.
b) An embolism is the displacement of solid, liquid, or gaseous particles by the bloodstream.

c) Cholesterol emboli usually affect the end arteries.
d) Arterial thrombosis is less common and more severe than arterial embolism.
e) In the upper extremity, arterial thrombosis as a cause of acute limb loss is very rare.

Answers

a) **Correct.** In most cases, about 80% of acute limb ischemias are due to embolic occlusion, and 20% to arterial thrombosis. For completeness, traumatic, iatrogenic, and malignant causes should also be mentioned, but these are absolute rarities.
b) **Correct.** Embolism is the displacement of particles, most often thrombi. The source of the latter is most often the heart (arrhythmia, ventricular aneurysm), but sometimes also upstream arteries (e.g., an aortic or popliteal aneurysm). Tumor tissue (atrial myxoma), amniotic fluid (during childbirth), fat, or air (both, for example, during fracture management) can also be carried by the bloodstream.
c) **Correct.** Cholesterol emboli usually arise in heavily calcified vessels (e.g., femoral bifurcation or femoropopliteal stenoses) and are typically carried into the end arteries. There, they cause very painful lesions, particularly affecting the acral regions.
d) **Incorrect.** Arterial thrombosis (about 20%) is much less common than embolism (about 80%) and, in most cases, is clinically less severe. This is due to the usually present collaterals that have developed over time.
e) **Correct.** Since PAD in the upper extremity is rare, arterial thrombosis in this location is also very rare. Acute occlusions in the shoulder and arm region are therefore most often embolic, but iatrogenic and traumatic causes are also not uncommon. Embolic occlusions in the upper extremity are often well compensated, due to naturally occurring collateral vessels. In clinical practice, decompensated ischemia in the upper extremity, which would present as livid discoloration, loss of sensorimotor function, or marked temperature difference, is rarely seen.

4. Which statements about Rudolf Virchow and his Virchow's triad are correct?

a) Virchow was a German vascular surgeon who studied blood coagulation intensively.
b) Virchow's triad includes changes in the vessel wall, blood composition, and flow characteristics.

c) Virchow also described an asthma triad.
d) Healthy endothelial cells have anticoagulant and fibrinolytic properties.
e) Virchow also studied leukemia.

Answers

a) **Incorrect.** Rudolf Ludwig Karl Virchow (1821–1902) was a German anatomist and pathologist who held a chair first in Würzburg and later in Berlin, and who studied blood coagulation and the development of thrombosis in depth.
b) **Correct.** As early as 1856, Virchow described in detail that the formation of blood clots in vessels is caused by changes in
   1. the vessel wall,
   2. the flow characteristics, and
   3. the blood composition

   The presence of any one of these three changes is sufficient to significantly increase the risk of thrombosis.
c) **Correct.** Since knowledge at that time was much less extensive than today, colleagues could work on many different topics. Among other things, Virchow also described the asthma triad, which is less well known than Virchow's triad in relation to thrombosis. The asthma triad describes the causes of bronchial obstruction, namely bronchospasm, hypersecretion, and edema/swelling.
d) **Correct.** Anticoagulant properties are mainly due to inhibition of platelets by prostaglandins and activation of fibrinolysis by expression of plasminogen activators. Conversely, pathophysiologically, defects in the endothelial layer, which are often seen in atherosclerosis, expose subendothelial vessel wall components, activating platelet aggregation via von Willebrand factor.
e) **Correct.** In his intensive study of tumors, including leukemia, Virchow discovered the increased tendency to clot in this disease, which was then called "white blood cancer," and gave it the name leukemia. He coined many other terms still in use today, such as glioma, sarcoma, myoma, embolism, and many more.

5. Which statements about compartment syndrome are correct?

a) Compartment syndrome describes the consequences of increased pressure in a compartment.
b) A compartment pressure of 15 mmHg is pathological and must be relieved by surgical opening of the compartment.

c) In severe ischemia (Rutherford II), 30–50% of patients develop manifest compartment syndrome after successful revascularization.
d) Prophylactic fasciotomy during surgical vascular revascularization of an acute occlusion should only be performed in exceptional cases.
e) Abdominal compartment syndrome is a typical complication of ruptured aortic aneurysm.

Answers

a) **Correct.** By definition, compartment syndrome involves an increase in pressure within a compartment surrounded by fascia or bone. If the function of tissue structures, especially arterial perfusion, is impaired as a result, the clinical signs of compartment syndrome develop.
b) **Incorrect.** Normal compartment pressure is 8–10 mmHg; at 30 mmHg, it is considered manifest compartment syndrome and should be relieved. For values between 10 and 30 mmHg, close monitoring and decongestive measures are recommended. In clinical practice, less reliance is placed on measured values and more on findings and the patient's subjective (and objectively verifiable) symptoms. If in doubt, it is better to indicate fasciotomy too early than too late.
c) **Correct.** The more severe the preoperative/interventional ischemic symptoms, the greater the risk of reperfusion syndrome. Local reperfusion syndrome corresponds to compartment syndrome, while systemic effects correspond to reperfusion syndrome. The latter typically presents as reddish urine (myoglobinuria) due to the breakdown of nonviable muscle.
d) **Incorrect.** Many surgeons perform prophylactic fasciotomy. This reduces the risk of delayed postoperative diagnosis and spares the patient a second procedure. If the surgeon initially decides to close the skin incision of the fasciotomy, the suture can be removed later (e.g., if tension increases in the ICU) without another anesthesia. The argument of an unnecessary skin wound is outweighed by the potential complications of delayed fasciotomy and subsequent limb loss.
e) **Correct.** In ruptured abdominal aortic aneurysm (rAAA), up to 30% of cases can develop abdominal compartment syndrome. This is especially true for endovascularly treated rAAA. Even with open repair, the abdominal wall sometimes cannot be closed primarily and must then be left open and sealed temporarily and sterilely (usually with a vacuum occlusive dressing). The prognosis for patients with an open abdomen after rAAA is significantly worse than after primary abdominal wall closure. However,

this is most likely due to the much worse initial situation with massive intra-abdominal blood loss (which is also the reason for the open abdomen), rather than the open abdominal wall itself.

6. Which statements about fasciotomy are correct?

a) Fasciotomy in young people should always be performed with the smallest possible incisions.
b) Fasciotomy of the lower leg is the most commonly performed technique in vascular surgery.
c) There are three compartments in the lower leg that must be opened during fasciotomy.
d) The risk of developing compartment syndrome after surgical/interventional vascular opening is 30–50%.
e) Prophylactic fasciotomy has proven effective in surgical vascular reconstruction (embolectomy, thrombectomy, bypass surgery).

Answers

a) **Incorrect.** In vascularly induced compartment syndrome, fasciotomy is generally not a cosmetic procedure but serves to preserve the limb. Therefore, skin incisions should be as large as necessary. Incisions that are too small, such as in semi-closed fasciotomy, jeopardize the surgical outcome.
b) **Correct.** Since about 90% of arterial occlusions involve the lower extremity, vascular (non-traumatic) compartment syndrome of the lower extremity is also much more common than in the upper extremity.
c) **Incorrect.** In fasciotomy of the lower leg, four compartments must be opened. These are:
   I. Anterior compartment
   II. Fibular (lateral) compartment
   III. Superficial flexor compartment
   IV. Deep flexor compartment

   A medial incision (for access to the flexor compartments) and a lateral incision (for access to the anterior and fibular compartments) have proven effective.
d) **Incorrect.** The risk of developing compartment syndrome is about 10–20% and depends, among other things, on the severity of preoperative ischemic symptoms. In decompensated ischemia (from Rutherford IIa), the risk increases sharply and can exceed 60%, whereas in stage I it is < 10%.

e) **Correct.** Many surgeons already open the compartments of the lower leg during vascular reconstruction by embolectomy/thrombectomy or bypass surgery and, if necessary, close the skin again. If compartment syndrome subsequently develops, the skin sutures can be removed without further surgery and the fascial wound can be covered with a VAC dressing. The consequences of delayed fasciotomy, which is not uncommon during on-call hours (outside regular working hours), are more serious and significant than the scars from prophylactic fasciotomy.

7. Which statements about ischemia tolerance are correct?

a) Ischemia tolerance is generally 6 hours.
b) Decompensated ischemia often occurs with occlusion of the femoral bifurcation.
c) In embolic occlusions, due to lack of collaterals, the 6-hour ischemia tolerance usually applies.
d) Cells of the nervous system have the lowest ischemia tolerance.
e) The ischemia tolerance of the small intestine is only 10–12 hours.

Answers

a) **False.** Ischemic tolerance always depends on the residual perfusion of the tissue. Complete ischemia without any residual perfusion is very rare. Usually, there is some residual perfusion, which is reflected in the clinical symptoms. Thus, the 6-hour rule does not fundamentally apply to every arterial occlusion. This applies in cases of (almost) complete ischemia, according to the Rutherford classification stage IIb.
b) **True.** Occlusions at the femoral bifurcation are often complete and lead to pronounced ischemia requiring urgent intervention within a maximum of 6 hours. Typically, the limb is cold and shows a complete sensorimotor deficit. Rapid development of a livid discoloration is also observed, which is a poor prognostic sign. This is frequently seen, for example, in elderly demented patients from nursing homes with an embolic occlusion of the femoral bifurcation.
c) **False.** Although embolic occlusions often result in more pronounced ischemia than arterial thrombosis due to insufficient collateralization, there are also regularly well-compensated arterial embolisms, for example, localized at the brachial bifurcation or the popliteal artery. This is due to often pre-existing natural collaterals (e.g., the genicular arteries at the level of the knee joint).

d) **True.** Nerve cells and brain tissue have a very low ischemic tolerance of only 2–4 hours, whereas muscle cells (6–8 hours) and skin (8–12 hours) are less sensitive. Even among nerve cells, there are gradations and differences in ischemic tolerance; brain cells are the most sensitive, followed by sensory nerve cells. Motor nerve fibers are less susceptible, primarily due to their thickness. This is also reflected in the clinical symptoms of acute ischemia: sensory nerve deficits are observed significantly before motor deficits, which is taken into account in the Rutherford classification (Rutherford IIa: sensory deficits, IIb: additionally motor deficits).

e) **False.** The intestine, especially the small intestine, is also among the tissues sensitive to ischemia with limited compensatory capacity, mainly because collaterals are only insufficiently developed. Consequently, bowel wall gangrene develops very quickly here, which externally appears as "black" bowel. Since the initial symptoms in acute mesenteric occlusion are often nonspecific and the bowel is difficult to assess externally, "mesenteric ischemia" is one of the most threatening acute arterial occlusions. Due to often delayed diagnosis and therapy, bowel wall perforation has already occurred in cases of extensive and irreversible ischemia.

8. Which statements about the Fogarty catheter are correct?

a) Thomas Fogarty was an American vascular surgeon who patented his invention of the balloon catheter in 1941 and manufactured it in his own company.

b) The Fogarty® catheter is available in different sizes and lengths, and the catheter tip is always configured the same way.

c) Embolectomy with a Fogarty catheter is an endovascular therapeutic procedure.

d) Embolectomy using the so-called "Fogarty maneuver" is minimally invasive with a low risk of complications.

e) The "thru-lumen" catheter is also suitable for infusion, aspiration of thrombi, and blood sampling.

Answers

a) **False.** Thomas Fogarty invented and patented the catheter named after him in 1963. At that time, he was in his surgical training and initially could not find a company willing to market his invention (which he had already used in numerous operations). He was not taken seriously by industrialists. His then-chief physician Al Starr therefore recommended the electrical engineer Lowell Edwards, who had his own small company (Edwards Life Sciences).

Edwards eventually began producing the catheters in 1969. From 1965, Fogarty published successful applications of his catheter.

b) **False.** There are different configurations of the catheter tip, depending on the area of application. The following catheter types can be obtained from Edwards Life Sciences:

I. Fogarty® arterial embolectomy catheter
   - for fresh arterial thrombi and embolism
   - Length 60/80 cm
   - Size 2–7 Fr
   - Diameter 4–14 mm

II. Fogarty® Fortis arterial embolectomy catheter
   - for older, partially organized emboli, stable balloon configuration allowing more force to be applied
   - Length 40/80 cm
   - Size 4 Fr
   - Diameter 8 mm

III. Fogarty® "thru lumen" embolectomy catheter
   - can be advanced over a wire, thus reducing vessel wall injuries
   - Length 40/80/ (120 for 3 Fr)
   - Sizes 3/4/5.5/6/7 Fr
   - Diameter 6–16 mm
   - Usable wires
     o 0.018: for all
     o 0.025: from 4 Fr
     o 0.035: from 5.5 Fr

IV. Fogarty® Corkscrew catheter
   - for older and difficult-to-remove clots
   - contains an extendable and retractable spiral at the tip
   - Length 40/80 cm
   - Sizes 4/5/6 Fr

V. Fogarty® graft thrombectomy catheter
   - for difficult-to-remove thrombi from bypasses and synthetic shunts
   - Length 50 cm
   - Sizes 5/6 Fr
   - Diameter 10–12 mm

VI. Fogarty® venous thrombectomy catheter
   - specifically for use in the venous system
   - has a long soft tip, which is intended to reduce the risk of injury to venous valves

- Length 80 cm
- Sizes 6/8 Fr
- Diameter 12–19 mm

VII. Fogarty® occlusion catheters

- specifically for intraluminal occlusion
- Lengths 40 (3–5 Fr) /80 cm (14 and 22 Fr)
- Sizes 3/4/5/14/22 Fr
- Diameter 6–45 mm

c) **True.** Strictly speaking, this is the first endovascular therapeutic procedure in combination with surgical exposure of an artery, thus a precursor to hybrid procedures.

d) **False.** With the "Fogarty maneuver," especially when performed by beginners, serious complications can indeed occur. These include, among others, dissection in the case of subintimal catheter placement, perforation, and rupture. Trainees should be thoroughly informed and sensitized to these risks. The use of a "thru-lumen" catheter, which is guided over a wire, should therefore be preferred, especially in the early stages, until a certain level of routine is achieved.

e) **True.** The "thru-lumen" catheter can be introduced over wires with a diameter of 0.018 inch, and from 5.5 French also over the commonly used 0.035 inch catheter. It also has barium markers proximal and distal to the balloon, which facilitates handling.

9. Which statements about Leriche syndrome are correct?

a) Leriche syndrome is fundamentally an acute event.

b) In high aortic occlusion (Leriche syndrome), there is a complete occlusion that begins above the renal arteries.

c) The mortality of acute Leriche syndrome is 50–80%.

d) Leriche syndrome is more often caused by arterial thrombosis than by embolism.

e) Radiological-interventional recanalization is the preferred procedure in acute high Leriche syndrome with limb ischemia according to Rutherford IIb.

Answers

a) **False.** Leriche syndrome (named after the French surgeon Rene Leriche) is an occlusion of the infrarenal aorta up to the bifurcation (or extending beyond), which can occur both acutely and chronically. Acute Leriche syndrome is a very serious condition with urgent surgical indication, usually with advanced ischemic symptoms. In the chronic form, symptoms of peripheral arterial disease (PAD) are observed, and there are also reports of erectile dysfunction, bladder and bowel emptying disorders (rectum!), and sometimes abdominal angina.

b) **False.** In high aortic occlusion according to Leriche, the occlusion begins directly infrarenally and extends to the aortic bifurcation or beyond. Acute occlusion is an emergency with urgent treatment indication and high mortality and lethality. In chronic high Leriche syndrome, there is often an extensive collateral network, so symptoms such as abdominal angina, erectile dysfunction, or buttock claudication are often reported.

c) **False.** The mortality of acute Leriche syndrome is indeed high, reported at 30–50%. The most common complications are postoperative renal failure due to reperfusion syndrome, especially in cases where temporary suprarenal clamping is necessary. Other complications include myocardial infarction, acute heart failure, and limb loss in cases of non-reconstructable or irreversible ischemia.

d) **True.** Acute Leriche syndrome is caused by arterial thrombosis and embolism in about half of cases each. In chronic Leriche syndrome, it is almost exclusively due to arterial thrombosis or progression of the underlying disease, atherosclerosis.

e) **False.** In high Leriche syndrome, surgical intervention should definitely be preferred to prevent shifting of the thrombus burden into the renal arteries. Moreover, only in stage I to IIa according to Rutherford would a usually more time-consuming interventional therapy be justified. In stage IIb, surgery is the treatment of choice. In addition to rapid restoration of arterial perfusion (by thrombectomy or bypass), fasciotomy of the lower leg of the affected limb should also be performed. In a decompensated perfusion situation (Rutherford IIb) and a high aortic occlusion, both systemic and local reperfusion syndrome must always be expected.

10. Which statements about intra-arterial lysis therapy are correct?

a) It is a minimally invasive procedure that should be preferred especially in elderly, pre-existing patients.

b) Monitoring should always take place in the intensive care or intermediate care unit.

c) rtPA (recombinant tissue plasminogen activator) is preferably used as a thrombolytic, alternatively urokinase.
d) Contraindications are known bleeding complications (cerebral hemorrhage, gastrointestinal bleeding, etc.), major surgery within the last 6 weeks, or Rutherford I ischemia.
e) Usually, a bolus is given (100–250 k IU urokinase or 5–10 mg Actilyse/rtPA/Alteplase), followed by continuous administration, which should always be weight-adapted.

Answers

a) **False.** Intra-arterial lysis therapy is often described as "minimally invasive" because it does not require a surgical approach. However, especially with increasing age, serious complications can occur, so the term "minimally invasive" is not entirely accurate. On the one hand, elderly patients benefit from the interventional approach, which can usually be performed under local anesthesia. On the other hand, elderly patients in particular, due to their comorbidities and sometimes fragile vessels, are prone to bleeding complications during lysis therapy, which can be life-threatening.
b) **True.** This is necessary to detect and respond to bleeding complications in a timely manner. Particular attention should be paid to sheath dislocations, which can be fatal on a general ward without monitor surveillance.
c) **True.** rtPA (recombinant tissue plasminogen activator) is now most commonly used, alternatively urokinase. Since 2019, there have been significant supply shortages of the latter, so in many hospitals almost exclusively rtPA (also available as Alteplase in Germany and Austria) was used. In 2022, the situation was reversed, as rtPA was temporarily unavailable due to the pandemic. Therefore, urokinase was primarily used in German hospitals. The guidelines of the SVS now advise against the previously frequently used streptokinase due to its high antigenic potential.
d) **False.** There are absolute and relative contraindications. The absolute contraindications commonly encountered in clinical practice include:
   I. **Rutherford IIb ischemia,** as no delay in revascularization can be tolerated here.
   II. **Rutherford III ischemia,** as this is a non-salvageable limb that should be amputated as soon as possible.

III. Manifest or impending **compartment syndrome,** where immediate surgical fasciotomy and arterial revascularization should be performed.
IV. Active or recent **bleeding complications** (< **10 days**, especially cerebral or gastrointestinal).
V. Recent **major surgical procedure** (**< 10 days**, e.g., laparotomy, endoprosthesis, craniotomy).
VI. Marked **non-compliance,** as there is a risk of sheath dislocation and bleeding both during the intervention and during subsequent lysis therapy.

A Rutherford I and IIa ischemia are not contraindications, nor is a surgical procedure with almost complete wound healing (provided there were no complications and the procedure was > 10 days ago). There are repeated situations where an interval of > 3 or even > 6 months from surgery is required. However, there is no evidence for this.

e) **False.** It is correct that usually a bolus (100,000 to 250,000 IU urokinase or 5–10 mg rtPA) is first administered into the thrombus. This is followed by continuous administration of the thrombolytic, either weight-adapted or according to a fixed protocol without weight adaptation. Numerous studies have shown no significant difference in efficacy between weight-adapted and non-weight-adapted protocols. Therefore, many hospitals use a standard protocol. It is important that the maximum dose of 40 mg rtPA should not be exceeded.
   - **Urokinase protocol:** 100,000–250,000 IU/h over 4h, then 50,000–150,000 IU/h for a maximum of 48h
   - **rtPA protocol:** 0.5–2.0 mg/h, maximum 40 mg

   Many working groups also recommend low-dose administration of unfractionated heparin via the sheath (500 IU/h) and additional peripheral heparin administration, which should be PTT-controlled (target 60–80 s).

11. Which statements about percutaneous aspiration thrombectomy (PAT) are correct?

a) PAT is an interventional procedure that can be used when lysis therapy is contraindicated.
b) The success rate of aspiration thrombectomy alone is over 90%.
c) Aspiration thrombectomy is an essential skill for interventional radiologists.
d) The Rotarex® S system is suitable for recanalization of chronic occlusions.
e) The Aspirex® S system is specifically designed for interventional recanalization of supra-aortic arteries.

Answers

a) **True.** PAT is an interventional procedure in which intra-arterial thrombi are aspirated and removed percutaneously. This procedure was first described by Starck in 1985 and has since been increasingly used in clinical practice. The principle is that a large-lumen, thin-walled catheter is advanced beyond the occlusion, and the thrombi are aspirated using a 50 ml syringe and removed via the sheath. To remove the thrombi at the catheter tip through the percutaneous access, sheaths with removable valves are used (e.g., Fortress® sheaths from Biotronik, size 5 or 6 French).
b) **False.** The success rate of aspiration thrombectomy alone in fresh arterial occlusions is about 30% if no other procedures are available or used. Combined with other interventional procedures such as mechanical aspiration, balloon angioplasty, and intra-arterial lysis therapy, the success rate is over 80%, which is comparable to surgical intervention.
c) **True.** The ability to perform aspiration thrombectomy is an indispensable technical skill for interventional radiologists. Especially during percutaneous interventions for chronic circulatory disorders, peripheral embolizations regularly occur, which should then be removed by aspiration thrombectomy.
d) **True.** The Rotarex® S system from Straub Medical can also be used to recanalize chronic occlusions, especially in-stent stenoses or occlusions. The principle of the catheter is that there are lateral openings at the tip through which thrombi and occlusion cylinders can be aspirated, reinforced by internal spirals that fragment and break up the material. However, caution is often required in native vessels, as the system can cause vessel wall injury. For recanalization of acute/subacute synthetic bypass occlusions or in-stent occlusions, however, it is usually very well suited.
e) **False.** The Aspirex® S system was specifically designed for recanalization of venous occlusions and thrombotic complications in hemodialysis shunts. The system is mainly capable of aspirating and fragmenting thrombi. The principle of detachment from the vessel wall is gentler than with the Rotarex® S system. Therefore, vessel wall injury is less common, but the system is less suitable for older occlusions.

12. Which statements about RCTs on acute limb ischemia are correct?

a) The ILAILL study investigated whether prostaglandins have a positive effect on mortality in acute limb ischemia.

b) The EUCLID study compared ticagrelor with clopidogrel medication in PAD patients.
c) Only patients with chronic, but not acute, circulatory disorders were included in the EUCLID study.
d) In acute limb ischemia, the endovascular approach is clearly superior to open surgery.
e) Both the VOYAGER-PAD and CASPAR studies showed that rivaroxaban significantly reduces the risk of acute ischemia after peripheral bypass surgery.

Answers

a) **Correct.** In the ILAILL study, almost 200 elderly patients (> 70 years) who had undergone surgery for acute limb ischemia were treated postoperatively for 7 days with either iloprost (Ilomedin®) or placebo. Allocation to each group was randomized and double-blind. Iloprost was administered intravenously daily for 4–7 days at a dose of approximately 70–100 ng/min (= 1-2 ampoules of 20 μg each) over 6 hours. The subsequent follow-up period was 90 days. The primary combined endpoint was mortality and amputation rate, with the risk in the placebo group being twice as high as in the prostaglandin group. Notably, almost one in three patients in the placebo group reached the primary endpoint, highlighting the severity of this disease and the multimorbidity of this patient population.
b) **Correct.** In the EUCLID study (Examining Use of Ticagrelor in Peripheral Artery Disease), the platelet function inhibitors ticagrelor and clopidogrel were compared in patients with PAD. No significant difference was found regarding cardiovascular (e.g., myocardial infarction) or limb-related (e.g., re-occlusion, amputation) complications.
c) **Incorrect.** The EUCLID study included patients with acute and chronic limb ischemia requiring inpatient treatment, who were randomized double-blind to the "ticagrelor" or "clopidogrel" group. Among the nearly 14,000 study patients, almost 2% (250 patients) had acute limb ischemia. When comparing these two subgroups (acute versus chronic), it was noted that
I. previous revascularizations,
II. atrial fibrillation,
III. an ankle-brachial index (ABI) < 0.6, and
IV. no prior statin medication
were significantly more common in patients with acute circulatory disorders. This is not surprising and is consistent with daily clinical experience.

What is surprising, however, is that patients with acute circulatory disorders were often younger than those with chronic PAD.
This does not correspond to the impression from daily clinical practice. This result could also be due to the fact that patients with acute ischemia at an advanced age are less frequently treated invasively, which was also one of the inclusion criteria.

d) **Incorrect.** In a 2015 meta-analysis[1] , which addressed precisely this question, it was shown that both procedures were equivalent regarding the endpoints of limb salvage and mortality after 30 days, 6 months, or 1 year. Strokes were more frequent after 30 days in the thrombolysis group at 1.3% compared to 0% in the surgical group (1.3% vs. 0%). The same applied to bleeding complications (8.8% versus 3.3%) and distal embolizations (12.4% versus 0%). However, these risks must be weighed against the individual surgical risk in each case. Consequently, based on the currently available evidence, no recommendations can be made for or against the endovascular or open approach.
e) **Incorrect.** In the VOYAGER-PAD study[2] (Vascular Outcomes Study of ASA Along With Rivaroxaban in Endovascular or Surgical Limb Revascularization for PAD), it was shown, among other things, that rivaroxaban 2.5 mg twice daily in combination with acetylsalicylic acid 100 mg once daily after surgical or endovascular peripheral revascularization offers a significant advantage over acetylsalicylic acid monotherapy. This applies to subsequent acute ischemia of the treated leg, cardiovascular complications (e.g., myocardial infarction, cardiovascular death), as well as limb loss.
In the CASPAR study (**C**lopidogrel and **A**cetylsalicylic Acid in Bypass **S**urgery for **P**eripheral **Ar**terial Disease), on the other hand, acetylsalicylic acid was compared with clopidogrel after peripheral bypass surgery. Here, no significant difference was found regarding subsequent acute ischemia,

[1] Branco BC, Montero-Baker MF, Mills JL Sr. The pros and cons of endovascular and open surgical treatments for patients with acute limb ischemia. J Cardiovasc Surg (Torino). 2015 Jun;56(3):401–7.

[2] Bonaca MP, Szarek M, Debus ES, Nehler MR, Patel MR, Anand SS, Muehlhofer E, Berkowitz SD, Haskell LP, Bauersachs RM. Efficacy and safety of rivaroxaban versus placebo after lower extremity bypass surgery: A post hoc analysis of a "CASPAR like" outcome from VOYAGER PAD. Clin Cardiol. 2022 Dec;45(12):1143–1146. https://doi.org/10.1002/clc.23926. Epub 2022 Oct 17. PMID: 36.251.249; PMCID: PMC9748742.

cardiovascular (myocardial infarction) or neurological (stroke), as well as limb-related (amputation) complications. However, after alloplastic bypass reconstruction, bypass occlusions occurred significantly less frequently, which is why the recommendation for dual antiplatelet therapy was concluded in this context.

In the initial results of the recently published "CASPAR-like" study, a post hoc analysis was performed to determine whether the "VOYAGER regimen" (acetylsalicylic acid with rivaroxaban versus acetylsalicylic acid monotherapy) offers advantages in a surgically treated cohort. There is evidence that rivaroxaban is beneficial here with regard to the CASPAR endpoints. Further studies and results are eagerly awaited.

13. Which statements about the 6 Ps according to Pratt are correct?

a) The 6 Ps according to Pratt are clinical signs of acute limb ischemia.
b) Prostration stands for shock and means something like complete exhaustion of the limb.
c) Gerald Hillary Pratt described and classified acute limb ischemia in more detail in 1954.
d) The coldness of the limb in arterial occlusion has no equivalent among the 6 Ps.
e) The livid discoloration occurs after the pallor (paleness), describes an improvement in the circulatory situation, and was therefore not described by Pratt.

Answers

a) **Correct**. The 6 Ps according to Pratt, often cited in the literature, are clinical signs of acute limb ischemia. They stand for:
   I. Pain
   II. Pulselessness
   III. Paleness
   IV. paresthesia
   V. paralysis
   VI. prostration
b) **Correct.** In contrast to systemic shock events (hypovolemic, cardiogenic, obstructive, or distributive), the term shock in acute limb occlusion vividly describes the complete exhaustion of the limb. Ultimately, the 6 Ps according to Pratt can also be classified according to the severity of the circulatory disorder. Pain, which can also be compensated or occur only with

exertion, is at the beginning, followed by pulselessness, pallor, then sensory disturbance, which occurs before motor impairment, and finally, as the maximal form of circulatory disorder, shock as complete loss of strength and movement of the limb.

c) **Correct.** Gerald Hillary Pratt was a cardiovascular surgeon from New York, who practiced, among other places, at Saint Vincent's Hospital. The Pratt test, which is used in addition to the Trendelenburg test to localize incompetent venous valves in varicosis, is also named after him. He also described the Pratt warning veins pretibially as the first sign of deep vein thrombosis of the leg. Despite his still significant contributions to vascular surgery, little is known about further details of his professional work and especially his private life. He lived from 1906–1979.

d) **Correct.** Strangely, the most important and prominent clinical feature, namely "the cold limb," is not listed among the classic 6 Ps. The 6 Ps stand for:

   I. Pain
   II. Paleness
   III. Pulselessness
   IV. Sensory and (paresthesia)
   V. motor impairment (paralysis), and
   VI. shock (prostration)

   The coldness is not specifically described or designated. The term **p**erishing (translated as extremely cold, bitterly cold) is sometimes used instead of **p**rostration. This can also serve as an aid for the often difficult-to-understand term prostration.

e) **Incorrect.** Pallor is the first skin sign of hypoperfusion and is caused, among other things, by vasoconstriction. If ischemia persists, the ratio of oxygenated to deoxygenated hemoglobin shifts, resulting in the livid discoloration. However, this is not described among the 6 Ps, even though it indicates progression of the circulatory disorder.

10 Non-atherosclerotic and Sports-associated Vascular Diseases

Question

1. Which statements about sports-associated vascular diseases are correct?

a) Iliac endofibrosis is one of the sports-associated stenosing arterial diseases.
b) Adductor canal syndrome is one of the sports-associated stenosing arterial diseases.
c) Cystic adventitial degeneration is one of the sports-associated stenosing arterial diseases.
d) Loeys-Dietz syndrome is one of the sports-associated stenosing arterial diseases.
e) Popliteal entrapment syndrome (PAES) is one of the sports-associated stenosing arterial diseases.

Answers

a) **Correct.** Iliac endofibrosis is a rare stenosing disease of the pelvic arteries, most commonly diagnosed in competitive cyclists and triathletes.
b) **Correct.** This refers to a stenosis of the superficial femoral artery at the level of the adductor canal, which is very rare and typically diagnosed in long-distance runners.
c) **Incorrect.** Cystic adventitial degeneration is characterized by cyst formation in the adventitia of the vessel wall, predominantly in the popliteal artery. It is most often diagnosed in men in their 40s to 50s, and a connection to athletic activity has not been described to date.

S. Regus, *Vascular Surgery: Questions and Answers*,
https://doi.org/10.1007/978-3-662-73387-5_10

d) **Incorrect.** Loeys-Dietz syndrome is an autosomal dominant connective tissue disorder that can be associated with palatal malformations (bifid uvula) and aortic aneurysms.
e) **Correct.** Functional PAES is caused by training-induced muscle hypertrophy in the popliteal fossa, resulting in compression of the artery.

Question

2. Which statements about popliteal entrapment syndrome (PAES) are correct?

a) It is a common disease.
b) It usually occurs in obese men in their 60s–70s.
c) The anatomical entrapment syndrome is classified into 6 types.
d) The functional entrapment syndrome is congenital.
e) The indication for surgical therapy should only be made in the event of complications.

Answers

a) **Incorrect.** It is a rare disease with an estimated incidence of 0.1–2% and fewer than 500 reported cases in the literature.
b) **Incorrect.** It is most often diagnosed in the 2nd–3rd decade of life, with a marked male predominance of 4:1.
c) **Correct.** PAES is classified into 6 types. In types 1–3, there is compression of the popliteal artery by the gastrocnemius muscle, which in type 2 inserts more laterally than normal, and in type 3 has accessory constricting muscle bands. In type 4, an abnormal course of the popliteus muscle is responsible for the compression. Type 5 involves both arterial compression and venous involvement. Type 6 describes the functional entrapment syndrome.
d) **Incorrect.** Functional PAES is a training-induced, and therefore acquired, hypertrophy of the calf muscles resulting in compression of the popliteal artery.
e) **Incorrect.** The indication for surgical therapy should be made upon diagnosis of abnormal knee joint anatomy, ideally before the onset of arterial complications. The goal is to remove the compressing muscle fibers without arterial reconstruction, which is only acceptable if the vessel wall is intact.

Question

3. Which statements about iliac endofibrosis are correct?

a) Iliac endofibrosis is a disease of advanced age.
b) Diagnosis is always made by MR angiography of the pelvic and leg arteries.
c) Clinical symptoms of iliac endofibrosis are exertional thigh and calf pain on the affected side.
d) There is no side preference.
e) Calcifications and atheromas in the affected arterial wall are histological features of iliac endofibrosis.

Answers

a) **Incorrect.** Iliac endofibrosis occurs predominantly in young athletes and is usually diagnosed in the 3rd–5th decade of life.
b) **Incorrect.** The most reliable diagnostic tool is measurement of the ankle-brachial Doppler index before and after maximal exertion. If it drops to 0.66 or less, the diagnosis of iliac endofibrosis is likely. Only then is MR angiography recommended for further therapy planning.
c) **Correct.** The typical symptoms occur during maximal training load or competition and are significantly performance-limiting.
d) **Incorrect.** In the majority of cases, the left side is affected. The reasons for this are unclear.
e) **Incorrect.** Calcifications and atheromas are typical findings in atherosclerosis. In iliac endofibrosis, there is an increase in connective tissue cells, especially fibroblasts and myeloblasts.

Question

4. What do you think of the following statements about adductor canal syndrome?

a) Adductor canal syndrome is the most common cause of thigh pain in long-distance runners.
b) The cause of adductor canal syndrome is repetitive compression of the artery at the level of the adductor canal.
c) Acute occlusion is the most common clinical presentation.

d) Recommendations for diagnosis and therapy have a low level of recommendation.
e) Stent PTA of the affected artery is the treatment of choice.

Answers

a) **Incorrect.** Adductor canal syndrome is a stenosing disease that occurs particularly in long-distance runners and long-distance triathletes, but it is a very rare cause of thigh pain. Much more common differential diagnoses include muscle fiber tears, overuse injuries, or stress fractures.
b) **Correct.** This mainly affects long-distance runners, especially since they tend to have highly developed thigh musculature and are subject to training-induced stress.
c) **Incorrect.** The most common symptom is exertional, unilateral calf pain. Acute occlusion, especially during competition, has also been described.
d) **Correct**. There are fewer than 30 publications worldwide on adductor canal syndrome, most of which are case reports. As a result, recommendations are based on expert opinion with an evidence level of C.
e) **Incorrect.** Once the diagnosis is made and if treatment is desired, surgical decompression should be performed, ideally before arterial damage occurs. Otherwise, in addition to dividing compressing muscle and tendon structures, arterial reconstruction may also be necessary.

Question

5. Which statements about cystic adventitial degeneration (CAD) are correct?

a) CAD is a disease of elderly people with a cardiovascular risk profile.
b) CAD is a rare arterial disease. There are only a few cases in the literature since its first description in 1947.
c) CAD is most commonly localized at the femoral bifurcation.
d) Histologically, it is characterized by cystic changes in the adventitia, which can lead to luminal narrowing.
e) CAD is usually treated conservatively.

Answers

a) **Incorrect.** Cystic adventitial degeneration (CAD) is a vascular disease that is most often diagnosed in the 3rd–5th decade of life. The etiology is not yet fully understood; several causes are suspected: on the one hand, a degenerative mucoid change due to microtrauma, and on the other, an origin in the joint capsule (supported by reports of occasional fistulous connections between the cystic changes and the joint capsule). A genetic cause due to the displacement of embryonic mucoid cells is also suspected.

b) **Correct.** CAD was first described in 1947 by Atkins and Key; interestingly, in this case the disease was localized in the external iliac artery, not the popliteal artery.
c) **Incorrect.** The main location is the popliteal artery, which is affected in over 85% of cases. This supports the theory that the cyst-forming cells originate in the joint and migrate or are displaced into the arterial wall via fistulous connections.
d) **Correct.** In CAD, cyst formation occurs in the arterial wall, predominantly in the adventitia, with increased fluid accumulation. Depending on the extent, this can result in progressive and significant narrowing of the vessel lumen. In the latter case, patients become symptomatic with claudication.
e) **Incorrect.** Since patients usually present with clinical symptoms and advanced disease at diagnosis, invasive therapeutic measures are recommended. There have been reports of successful cyst aspiration, but with rarely satisfactory long-term results. The latter is due to the persistence and progression of the disease, which is why surgical reconstruction should be indicated. The best long-term results are achieved with autologous reconstruction, such as interposition or patch repair.

Question

6. Which statements about thoracic outlet syndrome (TOS) are correct?

a) TOS can be anatomically divided into three groups.
b) TOS can be divided into three groups depending on the affected structure.
c) A cervical rib as a cause of TOS is more common in men than in women.
d) Gymnasts often have a scalenus syndrome due to muscle hypertrophy.
e) Hyperabduction syndrome is very rare.

Answers

a) **Correct.** Based on location and anatomical structures, TOS can be divided from proximal to distal into the following three syndromes:
   1. Scalenus syndrome
   2. Costoclavicular syndrome (most common)
   3. Hyperabduction syndrome.

Affected structures that can lead to potential neurovascular compression in these syndromes are, in the case of

1. Scalenus syndrome: the scalene muscles (scalenus anterior, medius, and posterior) as well as a cervical rib,
2. Costoclavicular syndrome: the clavicle and the first rib, and
3. Hyperabduction syndrome: the pectoralis minor muscle.

b) **Correct.** TOS is classified according to the compressed structures into neurological, arterial, and venous compression syndromes. The neurological compression syndrome is the most common (>95%), while the arterial and venous forms each account for about 1–3%.
c) **Incorrect.** Women are twice as likely as men to have a cervical rib. This may be one reason why about 70% of patients with TOS are female. The overall prevalence of a cervical rib is about 0.5–1%. Estimates suggest that cervical ribs become symptomatic in only 5–10% of cases, most commonly due to a compression syndrome.
d) **Incorrect.** There are no data showing an increased incidence of scalenus syndrome in gymnasts, even though they generally have training-induced hypertrophy of the neck and shoulder muscles. However, there are reports of non-union or unhealed fractures of the first rib in athletes who train and load the upper extremity, especially in ball sports such as handball, volleyball, or basketball, as well as gymnastics.
e) **Correct.** Hyperabduction syndrome is very rare and accounts for about 2–3% of TOS cases. Exact incidence figures are not available. Nevertheless, there is evidence that hyperabduction syndrome, as one of the three causes of TOS, occurs significantly more often in athletes than in non-athletes. This is due to the generally more prominent and training-induced hypertrophy of the upper extremity musculature, especially the pectoralis muscles.

Question

7. Which statements about nutcracker syndrome are correct?

a) Nutcracker syndrome is a compression-induced thrombosis of the left renal vein.
b) Nutcracker phenomenon and nutcracker syndrome are synonymous.
c) Typical symptoms of nutcracker syndrome usually only become apparent in advanced age.
d) The disease occurs more frequently in very slim young female patients.
e) The treatment of choice is venous stent implantation.

Answers

a) **Incorrect.** So-called nutcracker syndrome is a compression of the left renal vein between the abdominal aorta and the superior mesenteric artery. Thrombosis of the renal vein is extremely rare and is not a typical complication of nutcracker syndrome.
b) **Incorrect.** The term nutcracker **phenomenon** is used when compression of the renal vein is incidentally detected during investigations (e.g., ultrasound) but causes no clinical symptoms. In contrast, nutcracker **syndrome** is always associated with symptoms.
c) **Incorrect.** Typical symptoms of nutcracker syndrome usually occur in adolescents and young adults. Typical symptoms include left-sided lower abdominal and flank pain, macroscopic hematuria, severe menstrual pain, left-sided testicular pain, and a varicocele on the left side.
d) **Correct.** Very slim young women are much more frequently affected than normal- or overweight individuals. In addition, the disease is much more common in Asian countries and the Middle East than in Europe.
e) **Incorrect.** The treatment of choice is surgical intervention, with the best results achieved by reimplantation of the left renal vein into the inferior vena cava. This is now performed laparoscopically in most cases. There are also increasing reports of venous stent implantation, but with a high risk of recurrence and subsequent difficulty in surgical management if a stent is in place. Therefore, in young patients, a minimally invasive, laparoscopic reconstruction should be preferred.

Question

8. Which statements about Dunbar syndrome are correct?

a) Dunbar syndrome is a compression of the superior mesenteric artery by the renal vein.
b) A caudal course of the MAL at the level of the celiac trunk origin is extremely rare, observed in a maximum of 1% of the population.
c) Typical symptoms of Dunbar syndrome are nausea, vomiting, and cramp-like epigastric pain after eating.
d) The treatment of choice for Dunbar syndrome is laparoscopic division of the MAL.
e) Abdominal angina and Dunbar syndrome describe the same clinical entity.

Answers

a) **Incorrect.** In Dunbar syndrome, there is compression of the celiac trunk (CT) by the median arcuate ligament (MAL). This ligament connects the two crura of the diaphragm, right and left, both of which normally originate from the 12th thoracic vertebra and between which the aorta passes. The MAL runs ventral to the aorta and usually several centimeters above the CT. However, in cases of an unusually caudal course, it can also compress the CT, which is then described as Dunbar syndrome. In English-language literature, it is often referred to as MALS (median arcuate ligament syndrome). Dunbar syndrome was first described in 1917 by Benjamin Lipshutz, and then in detail in 1965 by Dunbar and Marable.[1]

b) **Incorrect.** Although the ligament normally runs several centimeters above the CT ventral to the aorta, up to 25% of people have a caudal course at the level of the CT. This inevitably leads, especially during deep inspiration, to compression of the CT. However, only about 1% of people with a caudal MAL course develop symptoms, making the condition very rare.

c) **Correct.** The classic triad of Dunbar syndrome includes epigastric pain, weight loss, and an audible bruit on auscultation.

d) **Incorrect.** Although laparoscopic division of the ligament is possible in principle, the open approach is preferred. Especially if reconstruction of the CT is necessary, laparotomy is definitely indicated. Interventional therapy with stent-supported PTA is also possible and sometimes successful, but with a high risk of recurrence. Simple PTA without stenting is not recommended, as it is generally unsuccessful.

e) **Incorrect.** In abdominal angina, there is typically a narrowing or occlusion of the SMA, whereas in Dunbar syndrome, the CT is affected. However, there is often overlap between the two conditions, especially in abdominal angina. If the SMA is stenosed or occluded and is also compressed by the MAL, the symptoms of SMA stenosis can be much more pronounced than without CT compression. Conversely, an asymptomatic patient with a caudal MAL course may develop symptoms if there is additional flow impairment of the SMA. However, SMA compression as part of Dunbar syndrome does not normally occur.

---

[1] Dunbar JD, Molnar W, Beman FF, Marable SA. Compression of the celiac trunk and abdominal angina. Am J Roentgenol Radium Ther Nucl Med. 1965 Nov;95(3):731–44. https://doi.org/10.2214/ajr.95.3.731. PMID: 5844938.

Question

9. Which statements about pelvic congestion syndrome (PCS) are correct?

a) Pelvic congestion syndrome (PCS) is also called ovarian insufficiency.
b) PCS is a rare cause of chronic lower abdominal pain in women.
c) PCS is always bilateral.
d) In women with known varicose veins in the legs and chronic lower abdominal pain, PCS should be considered as a differential diagnosis.
e) The treatment of choice for PCS is embolization of the affected ovarian veins.

Answers

a) **Correct.** PCS is also called ovarian vein insufficiency, as it is caused by congestion and dilation of the pelvic veins and is observed mainly in women. A corresponding equivalent in men has not been described or does not have its own designation.
b) **Incorrect.** After endometriosis (about 10% of women are affected), PCS is the second most common cause of chronic lower abdominal pain in women: approximately 5% are affected by PCS. The symptoms of both conditions are similar, typically lower abdominal pain and pain during or after intercourse. The most important difference is the cycle dependency in endometriosis, which does not exist in PCS. Conservative medical therapy is also similar and primarily symptomatic, namely:
   1. Combined oral contraceptives
   2. Progestins
   3. Danazol
   4. NSAIDs
   5. GnRH analogues
c) **Incorrect.** PCS can also be localized unilaterally, for example in the context of the so-called nutcracker syndrome. In this condition, the left renal vein is compressed between the aorta and the superior mesenteric artery. As a result, thrombosis, outflow obstruction, or varicosis due to valve insufficiency of the left ovarian vein may occur. This vein normally drains into the left renal vein. In most cases, however, PCS is localized bilaterally.
d) **Correct.** More than 50% of women suffering from PCS also have concomitant varicosis in the legs. There is evidently a certain genetic predisposition to varicose vein disease, not only in the extremities but also in the abdomen or pelvis.

e) **Correct.** Interventional treatment has now become established, as it offers many advantages compared to open surgery. The following materials are used for radiological-interventional occlusion:
   1. Coils (mostly made of nickel)
   2. Plugs
   3. Sclerosing agents (Aethoxysklerol® = polidocanol)

Traumatic Vascular Injuries

11

Question

1. Which statements regarding the classification of traumatic vascular injuries are correct?

a) The classification of traumatic vascular injuries can be divided into sharp and blunt injuries.
b) A traumatic vascular injury is always recognizable by a bleeding complication.
c) Traumatic vascular injuries can be classified into arterial and venous injuries.
d) There are primary and secondary traumatic vascular injuries.
e) There are three degrees of severity of traumatic vascular injuries.

Answers

a) **Correct.** Traumatic vascular injuries are often classified according to their mechanism of origin into sharp and blunt injuries. In sharp injuries, the adventitia is usually affected first, before the injury (depending on the severity and extent of the trauma) extends from the outside inwards. In blunt trauma, it is the opposite: here, the intima is injured first (dissection), after which the injury extends from the inside outwards into the media and adventitia.
b) **Incorrect.** Traumatic vascular injuries do not necessarily lead to bleeding complications. This can be explained by the often intact adventitia (and sometimes media) in blunt injuries, as well as the retraction of the vessel

S. Regus, *Vascular Surgery: Questions and Answers*,
https://doi.org/10.1007/978-3-662-73387-5_11

ends in complete (sharp or blunt) transection. Consequently, ischemia is more often the first sign of a traumatic vascular injury than bleeding.

c) **Correct.** Approximately 80% of traumatic vascular injuries affect arteries. Veins are affected in only about 10–20% of cases, and then rarely in isolation. Arterial injuries can lead to life-threatening bleeding, which is why they are particularly feared. However, venous injuries should not be underestimated: they too can lead to life-threatening events, especially since the bleeding is often not recognized for a longer period and venous vessels do not invert or invert less than arterial vessels. Intraoperative iatrogenic venous injuries, especially to the iliac or caval veins, are often more difficult to manage than arterial injuries.
d) **Correct.** Primary vascular lesions are the immediate result of trauma, such as intimal lesions, dissections, or total/subtotal disruptions of continuity. Secondary vascular injuries include aneurysms, which are caused by reduced wall stability or elasticity. Unrecognized injuries can also lead to aneurysm formation, often in the form of a false aneurysm.
e) **Correct.** At least according to Vollmar, both sharp and blunt vascular injuries can be classified into three degrees of severity:

- **sharp** (according to extension from outside to inside):
  1. Adventitia
  2. Media
  3. Intima
- **blunt** (according to extension from inside to outside):
  1. Intima
  2. Media
  3. Adventitia

Question

2. Which statements regarding the diagnosis of traumatic vascular injuries are correct?

a) A traumatic vascular injury is easily diagnosed by ischemia.
b) If a popliteal artery injury is suspected in a knee dislocation fracture, angiography should be performed as soon as possible.
c) In young patients, magnetic resonance angiography (MRA) should be preferred over CTA for further diagnosis of traumatic vascular injuries.

d) If a traumatic injury of the thoracic aorta is suspected in a hemodynamically unstable pregnant woman, an emergency CTA is indicated despite radiation exposure.
e) If, after surgical treatment of an elbow dislocation fracture, one hand is noticeably cooler compared to the other, the pulse status should first be assessed and an ultrasound performed.

Answers

a) **Incorrect.** A traumatic vascular injury can easily be overlooked, even if a major vessel is involved. This is partly due to the often severe osseous injuries, which are the focus in the emergency department. In addition, collateral vessels are often present, maintaining peripheral perfusion (for example, in the popliteal or brachial artery) and masking ischemia. Therefore, in extremity injuries resulting from high-energy trauma (such as knee dislocation), the pulse status should always be assessed during the initial examination.
b) **Incorrect.** If a traumatic arterial vascular injury is suspected, a CT angiography (CTA) should be performed as soon as possible. The advantages of CTA are that the examination can be performed within a few minutes and allows assessment of both the vessel lumen and the vessel wall as well as the surrounding tissue.
c) **Incorrect.** In emergencies, MRA has the significant disadvantage that the examination takes much longer than CTA and the vessel wall can only be inadequately assessed. Artifacts are also common, especially when temporary immobilization devices have been applied after reduction. Therefore, the disadvantages of contrast agent and radiation exposure should be accepted in order to quickly obtain a reliable diagnosis based on meaningful imaging.
d) **Correct.** In an emergency, everything must be done to protect the patient's life. Failure to treat a traumatic aortic rupture in a pregnant woman also endangers the life of the unborn child, so everything must be done to stop the bleeding. In a hemodynamically unstable woman, CTA is the fastest way to secure the diagnosis and plan therapy.
e) **Correct.** Before performing CTA, MRA, or even DSA, the pulse status of both the affected and unaffected side should first be assessed. If a pulse deficit is detected, duplex sonography is recommended. Only if abnormal findings (vessel interruption, hematomas, monophasic distal flow profiles)

are found should further diagnostics be pursued. Often, the sonographic finding alone is sufficient to plan further surgical or interventional therapy. If there is a complete interruption of the vessel lumen, suspicion of arterial avulsion is present, necessitating surgical intervention.

Question

3. Which statements regarding traumatic carotid dissection are correct?

a) Dissections of extracranial brain-supplying arteries are among the main causes of ischemic stroke in young adults.
b) Traumatic carotid dissection is rare in young people without pre-existing conditions and occurs in < 1% of polytraumatized patients.
c) A typical accident mechanism that should prompt consideration of carotid dissection is high-velocity trauma with a helmet in place.
d) Traumatic dissection of extracranial brain-supplying arteries is associated with a high stroke risk of over 20%.
e) In traumatic dissection of the ICA, permanent oral anticoagulation for at least 6 months is indicated.

Answers

a) **Correct.** Dissections of the extracranial internal carotid and vertebral arteries are among the main causes of ischemic stroke in young adults. Their annual incidence is about 2–3/100,000 each, with a high number of unreported cases assumed. In addition to traumatic dissections, there are also spontaneous and those associated with aortic dissections.
b) **Incorrect.** Traumatic carotid dissection is indeed very rare, but still occurs in about 5% of polytrauma patients. It is often overlooked or only noticed later during inpatient treatment. Early diagnosis, however, can help prevent ischemic events. Therefore, in every polytrauma patient, and especially in cases of cervical spine trauma, further diagnostics to rule out carotid dissection are recommended.
c) **Correct.** High-velocity trauma with a helmet in place, especially in motorcyclists, is the most common cause of traumatic carotid dissections and is often overlooked, as it is initially clinically silent and unimpressive. Therefore, such accident mechanisms accompanied by hematomas of the neck soft tissues should always prompt consideration of traumatic carotid dissection and further diagnostics.

d) **Incorrect.** The stroke risk of traumatic dissection of extracranial brain-supplying arteries is only about 5–7%. Nevertheless, early recognition is extremely important to prevent a potentially life-threatening or disabling stroke. Initial therapy focuses on heparin administration, followed by antiplatelet therapy and blood pressure control.
e) **Incorrect.** There is evidence that initial anticoagulation with heparin leads to significantly better outcomes and, in particular, reduces the number of ischemic events. However, prolonged oral anticoagulation over several months is generally not indicated. The bleeding risk and further extension of a mural hematoma, as well as the potential benefit of recanalization, should always be weighed. Heparin administration in the initial phase and subsequent antiplatelet therapy (APT) are standard treatments, but there is no consensus among experts regarding the duration of APT, and practices vary.

Question

4. Which statements regarding traumatic extremity amputation are correct?

a) About 5% of major amputations are due to trauma.
b) The level of amputation should be as distal as possible.
c) The most common cause of traumatic amputations is traffic accidents.
d) In traumatic vascular injuries as the cause of limb loss, transfer time to the nearest hospital is the most important factor for the level of amputation.
e) Phantom pain is rare after traumatic amputations.

Answers

a) **Correct.** At most, 5% of major amputations are due to trauma, whereas the majority of amputations (80%) are due to peripheral arterial occlusive disease (PAOD). Of these, 70% are a consequence of diabetes mellitus. Tumor diseases also account for less than 5%.
b) **Correct.** In principle, the level of amputation should be as distal as possible in every case. This is especially true for traumatic amputations, as these usually affect young patients. Mobilization with a prosthesis is crucial for patients and their quality of life, but prosthetic suitability should also be considered when making the indication. The basic principle "as little as possible" also includes "as much as necessary," so necrotic, nonviable, and non-load-bearing tissue should never be left behind. The revision rate for traumatic amputations is about 25–30%, higher than in PAOD patients.

This may be due to the much greater motivation to preserve a long stump in young patients.

c) **Incorrect.** The most common cause of traumatic amputations is sports and leisure accidents, accounting for about 35–40%. Traffic accidents are much less common and are responsible for only about 25–30% of traumatic amputations. The third most common cause is occupational accidents.
d) **Incorrect.** Studies have shown that transfer time to the nearest hospital (as long as it remains within 20–60 minutes) has no influence on the likelihood of limb loss or the level of amputation itself.
e) **Incorrect.** Phantom pain is very common after traumatic amputations, especially in upper extremity amputations. Here, 40–80% of patients report corresponding neurogenic complaints, so surgical revision is by no means rare. Interestingly, phantom pain and neuromas are much more common after amputations of the dominant arm than the non-dominant arm. This may be due to preoperative baseline anatomy, but also to greater postoperative use and strain.

Question

5. Which statements regarding traumatic injury of the popliteal artery are correct?

a) Traumatic injury of the popliteal artery most commonly occurs in stab wounds.
b) Clinically, an avulsion injury of the popliteal artery always presents with a progressively enlarging hematoma and manifest compartment syndrome.
c) Definitive osteosynthetic management of the osseous injury is the main priority.
d) Fasciotomy is not recommended in these often young patients without cardiovascular risk factors.
e) According to current evidence, postoperative oral anticoagulation or antiplatelet therapy must be administered permanently.

Answers

a) **Incorrect.** Injury to the popliteal artery often occurs with blunt trauma, particularly with knee dislocation or fracture-dislocation. A typical mechanism is a dislocation injury with massive force.
b) **Incorrect.** Clinically, peripheral circulatory disturbance with pulse and possibly sensorimotor deficit is the main feature. Because the severed

artery retracts and inverts at both ends, the accompanying hematoma is often surprisingly small.

c) **Incorrect.** Prompt reduction of the fracture and stabilization of the joint position are important. Application of an external fixator is recommended (time required should be kept to 15–30 minutes). As soon as possible, surgical management and restoration of arterial perfusion should follow. Definitive and time-consuming osteosynthesis should be performed later.
d) **Incorrect.** Fasciotomy with generous and consistent opening of all four compartments should always be performed to avoid missing the frequently postoperative compartment syndrome and thus prevent irreversible tissue damage or major amputation.
e) **Incorrect.** After reconstruction of a traumatic arterial injury, most authors recommend administration of an antiplatelet agent (APA) for about 3–12 months, although there is no clear evidence for this. Interestingly, a meta-analysis found no significant differences in immediate occlusion rates between patient groups who received only APA and those who received therapeutic heparin in the immediate postoperative phase (days 1–5).

Question

6. Which statements regarding traumatic injury of the axillary artery are correct?

a) The axillary artery is very well protected in the axillary soft tissue, and traumatic injury is therefore rare.
b) Clinically, injury to the axillary artery always presents with acute hand ischemia.
c) If axillary artery avulsion is suspected, angiography with interventional readiness is the diagnostic method of choice.
d) For surgical management of the axillary artery, ipsilateral arm positioning and sterile draping of a thigh are recommended.
e) The amputation risk in axillary artery injuries is very high and is 30–50%.

Answers

a) **Incorrect.** After the brachial (cubital) artery, the axillary artery is the most commonly affected by traumatic injuries of the arteries in the upper extremity. Sharp injuries are rare, but most are blunt injuries following significant force with humeral fractures and shoulder dislocations.

b) **Incorrect.** Due to good collateral circulation (thoracoacromial artery, subscapular artery, and posterior and anterior circumflex humeral arteries), ischemic symptoms are often only mild to moderate (Rutherford I to IIa).
c) **Incorrect.** The diagnostic method of choice is now CT angiography. Its advantages are clear: it is a noninvasive examination, can be performed within a few minutes, and allows reliable assessment of perfusion, vessel continuity, and paravascular hematoma.
d) **Correct.** The arm should be positioned or at least movable to allow exploration in both abduction and adduction. Sterile draping of a thigh is often forgotten but can be very helpful for autologous reconstruction. The arm veins are often involved and are unsuitable as graft material.
e) **Incorrect.** The amputation risk is very low. Amputation of the hand or forearm is usually only indicated if the soft tissue damage is extensive and limb salvage cannot be ensured. The ischemia-related amputation rate is low and is less than 5%.

Question

7. Which statements regarding traumatic avulsion of the brachial artery are correct?

a) Traumatic injury of the brachial (cubital) artery most commonly occurs with elbow dislocation or fracture-dislocation.
b) Patients with traumatic avulsion of the brachial artery often present with pronounced ischemic symptoms.
c) Patients with traumatic avulsion of the brachial artery are usually middle-aged men.
d) In most cases, a traumatically injured brachial artery must be replaced with an alloplastic interposition graft.
e) In children, the anastomosis should be performed using interrupted technique with absorbable suture material.

Answers

a) **Correct.** Typically, elbow dislocation or fracture-dislocation can result in avulsion of the brachial artery at the level of the elbow (often referred to as the cubital artery in clinical practice).
b) **Incorrect.** Ischemic symptoms are usually very well compensated; an absent radial pulse on clinical examination is often the key finding.

c) **Incorrect.** It often occurs in children, in whom a supracondylar humerus (dislocation) fracture results in partial or complete transection of the brachial artery.
d) **Incorrect.** Ideally, if the posterior wall is partially preserved, the artery can be patched autologously. In complete transection, an interposition graft is usually required. The great saphenous vein (GSV) or alternatively the basilic vein is most commonly used. Due to poor patency rates and increased infection risk in potentially contaminated surgical fields, the use of alloplastic materials is strongly discouraged.
e) **Correct.** In children, absorbable suture materials in interrupted technique are recommended to prevent circumferential stenosis of the anastomosis region in adulthood as the organism grows.

Question

8. Which general statements regarding the surgical management of traumatically injured or occluded vessels are correct?

a) Most sharp injuries can be repaired by direct suture.
b) Traumatically induced dissections of the carotid artery can usually be managed conservatively.
c) In Paget-von-Schrötter syndrome, invasive therapy must be performed immediately.
d) Penetrating foreign bodies (knife, stake, etc.) should be removed immediately to minimize blood loss as much as possible.
e) Primary fasciotomy should be performed not only at the level of the vascular injury but also distally.

Answers

a) **False.** In most cases, even a sharp injury cannot be directly sutured, as the surrounding damage to the vessel is too extensive. In addition, the retraction force of the vessel causes the cut edges to pull apart, making direct suturing even more difficult.
b) **Correct.** Traumatic dissections of the carotid artery occur, for example, in whiplash injuries or suicide attempts by hanging. These can often be treated conservatively, and interventional therapy is rarely necessary. In the event of complications such as thrombotic occlusion, local thrombolysis is usually performed, followed by stenting of the dissection. The occurrence

of specific neurological deficits in the sense of a TIA or stroke must also prompt a strict evaluation of the indication for available invasive measures.

c) **False.** Paget-von-Schroetter syndrome is an acute thrombosis of the subclavian or axillary vein, usually triggered by exertion. For this reason, it is also called "effort thrombosis." The management of thrombosis in the context of Paget-von-Schroetter syndrome is generally conservative, using compression therapy and anticoagulation as well as symptomatic pain management. Surgical thrombectomy is rarely indicated, and would be considered, for example, if the superior vena cava is involved and there is a risk of venous embolism due to continued inflow from the contralateral side. In addition, anatomical causes such as cervical ribs or narrowing of the thoracic outlet should be ruled out.
d) **False.** Penetrating foreign bodies in the extremities, and especially in the thorax or abdomen, should never be removed on site. This can lead to acute exsanguination if major vessels have been injured. Removal of large penetrating foreign bodies should only be performed in the hospital, preferably under sterile conditions in the operating room.
e) **Correct.** Fasciotomy is generally indicated and should be performed generously. The fascia should be opened not only at the level of the vascular injury but also distally. At the site of the vascular injury, tissue swelling occurs, particularly due to bleeding and hematoma. Distal to the vascular injury, swelling typically occurs due to arterial reperfusion, which is more pronounced the longer the ischemia has persisted.

Question

9. Which statement about the reconstruction of traumatically damaged arteries is correct?

a) A complete replacement of traumatically injured arteries is rarely necessary.
b) For autologous replacement of a ruptured popliteal artery, the popliteal vein is ideally suited and is located nearby.
c) In the case of completely transected arteries of a limb, a shunt should, if possible, be inserted at the accident site.
d) In the case of transection of the common carotid artery, an 8 mm PTFE interposition graft is better than the great saphenous vein.
e) In war zones (e.g., Ukraine war), human acellular prostheses are an alternative to autologous grafts.

Answers

a) **False.** In the case of complete transection of an artery, a full replacement is generally required. This is also due to the behavior of the artery after complete transection. The ends of the severed artery retract and invert to stop the bleeding. Therefore, the arterial ends must be trimmed to provide a suitable bed for the anastomosis. However, direct reanastomosis would place the suture under too much tension, so an interposition graft should be inserted. This should be autologous whenever possible.

b) **False.** The popliteal vein is not the preferred vessel for replacing a ruptured popliteal artery, which usually occurs in the context of knee dislocation. On the one hand, it is also frequently injured, sometimes even transected. On the other hand, its wall is very thin and often develops aneurysms over time. For this reason, harvesting the great saphenous vein from the thigh is recommended. The great saphenous vein at the level of the knee joint can also be harvested, but it is often too small in diameter to be suitable as a replacement. This should be considered when draping the surgical field to ensure sterile access to the great saphenous vein up to the saphenofemoral junction if needed.

c) **False.** Placement of an intraluminal shunt is rarely possible or necessary directly at the accident site. Only in exceptional cases, when both ends are already externally visible, can this be attempted. However, the procedure requires a certain level of expertise, is time-consuming, and carries a significant risk of peripheral embolization and infection. For this reason, ideally, no time should be lost and the patient should be transferred directly to the nearest hospital with vascular surgical expertise.

d) **False.** Even if the common carotid artery needs to be reconstructed, an autologous interposition graft should be preferred in traumatic injuries. If, however, the great saphenous vein has a diameter of less than 2 mm or is otherwise unsuitable or absent, a segment of the common or superficial femoral artery can be harvested and used for reconstruction of the common carotid artery. Subsequently, the harvested femoral artery is reconstructed, and a PTFE interposition graft can be used here. The use of PTFE in a potentially contaminated trauma field should, however, be strictly avoided.

e) **Correct.** Human Acellular Vessels (HAV) are a very promising biological vascular substitute developed by Humacyte®, which is particularly successful in shunt surgery for dialysis patients. However, these grafts can also be used for peripheral vascular replacement and in infection-prone areas. Approval has not yet been granted. Nevertheless, their use can be justified in emergency situations, especially in war scenarios. These prostheses, made from human tissues and subsequently "decellularized," are, like PTFE prostheses, available in standard diameters and lengths (usually 6 mm in diameter and 20–40 centimeters in length), can be stored, and are thus quickly available when needed. This allows the operation time for polytraumatized patients to be kept as short as possible. These prostheses are plastic-free and therefore significantly less susceptible to infection, which is very important and decisive for limb salvage in traumatic and especially war-related injuries.

Question

10. Which statement about the behavior of traumatically damaged arteries is correct?

a) Traumatically transected arterial ends are generally very close together and easily adaptable.
b) Tying off the limb is important, as this is the only way to stop the bleeding.
c) Sometimes a local intimal lesion and dissection leads to occlusion, but continuity is preserved.
d) Atherosclerotically altered vessels rarely rupture completely, as the vessel wall is more stable and resistant due to calcifications.
e) Traumatic vascular injuries in childhood are almost never seen due to the elasticity of the arteries.

Answers

a) **False.** Both sharply and bluntly transected arteries generally retract and are usually several centimeters apart. In addition, the ends of the arteries are often so badly lacerated that trimming of the edges is necessary. For this reason, reconstruction using an interposition graft is often required.
b) **False.** The so-called tourniquet maneuver, with application of a tourniquet proximal to the bleeding source and compression above systolic blood pressure, has a justified place in emergency medicine. Nevertheless, the body can help itself through a special mechanism to stop the bleeding. The severed arterial ends invert, and a thrombus usually forms there, closing the artery at both ends.
c) **Correct.** Blunt trauma and distortions can cause an isolated intimal lesion, leading to vessel occlusion. In CT imaging, the vessel wall appears continuous, but there is no luminal perfusion. The treatment of choice is partial intimal resection, refixation, and autologous patch plasty. Alterna-

tively, interventional treatment with balloon angioplasty and, if necessary, stent implantation can be performed.

d) **False.** Calcified vessels in the presence of concomitant peripheral arterial disease can also rupture completely due to trauma. However, they are more prone to dissections and plaque tears, which can make interventional treatment more difficult. Open reconstruction is also generally more challenging than in healthy vessels.
e) **False.** Children's arteries can also dissect and rupture, typically in severely displaced supracondylar humerus fractures. The vessel ends can become trapped in the fracture gap and are easily overlooked. Complicating matters, pediatric patients often do not express ischemic symptoms. It is therefore all the more important to carefully assess pulse status, sensorimotor function, and capillary refill preoperatively, and to contact vascular surgery early.

Question

11. Which statements about compartment syndrome after traumatic vascular injuries are correct?

a) In the case of traumatic transection of the popliteal artery, a fasciotomy should be performed on the lower leg.
b) A distinction is made between traumatic and non-traumatic compartment syndrome.
c) In fasciotomy during reconstruction of an occluded popliteal artery, the tibial nerve should be decompressed.
d) A fasciotomy of the upper or lower arm is only necessary in exceptional cases after traumatic avulsion of the axillary artery.
e) A so-called "second look" after fasciotomy should be performed after 48 hours.

Answers

a) **Correct.** Because avulsion of the popliteal artery (i.e., complete transection) often leads to inadequately compensated perfusion due to poor collateralization, fasciotomy is strongly recommended. This should be generously indicated even if the musculature appears normal and there is only slight tension during the initial procedure. Otherwise, despite successful revascularization, limb loss may occur if fasciotomy is not performed or is delayed.
b) **Correct.** Compartment syndrome is classified as traumatic (strictly speaking, without injury to a major vessel and without ischemia) or non-traumatic

(the classic reperfusion syndrome after revascularization of an acute arterial occlusion, which was caused by arterial thrombosis or embolism). In traumatic vascular injury, however, there is regularly a combination of both entities, so clinical distinction is hardly possible and also irrelevant. Traumatic compartment syndrome arises primarily due to increased tension in the compartment from bleeding and hematoma formation.

c) **Correct.** The tibial nerve often becomes entrapped in the fascial arch of the gastrocnemius muscle during traumatic popliteal artery avulsion, which can result in irreversible nerve damage despite successful fasciotomy. Complete loss of limb function may also occur.
d) **False.** Compartment syndrome can also occur in the arm and must be relieved in a timely manner. It is much less common than in the lower leg, probably due to less well-developed musculature. Good collateralization, which is usually present, is also often the reason for the rare occurrence of reperfusion problems in the arm after arterial occlusions. However, after traumatic events, fasciotomy is regularly necessary and should include splitting of the carpal tunnel. On the volar forearm, the skin incision is curved, and dorsally it is straight. Complete opening of the flexor compartments is important, which can be achieved with a straight fasciotomy. The skin incision is curved volarly to minimize functional limitations from inevitable scarring and contractures, which are much less pronounced with a curved incision than with a straight one.
e) **Correct.** The recommendation is to perform the first "second look" 48 hours after the initial fasciotomy. The rationale is that necrotic muscle areas can then be removed and no longer harm the systemic circulation. If there are already tension-free and unremarkable soft tissue and skin conditions, secondary closure should be performed. If further dressing changes are necessary, vacuum sealing is recommended; the next dressing change can then be performed after 48–96 hours (provided the wound conditions are unremarkable).

Question

12. What is the significance of pulse status in the initial examination of polytraumatized patients?

a) Palpable foot pulses in polytraumatized patients rule out acute ischemia.
b) Weakly palpable foot pulses in polytraumatized patients are proof of an arterial lesion.

c) Determination of the ankle-brachial index (ABI) is important in peripheral arterial disease, but not in suspected traumatic vascular injury.
d) If an unremarkable pulse status is documented during the initial examination, further checks of perfusion are not necessary.
e) The initial examination of pulse status in polytrauma patients can be complicated by constrictive dressings.

Answers

a) **False.** Even with palpable foot pulses, arterial lesions, especially intimal lesions in the form of dissections, may be present. In addition, it is not uncommon for first responders, due to lack of experience and the hectic environment at the accident site or in the trauma bay, to feel their own pulse. They then give a "false all-clear," and the risk of missing a vascular injury is high.
b) **False.** Weakly palpable foot pulses may, in the hands of an experienced examiner, be a strong indication of an arterial lesion, but they are by no means proof. Especially bilaterally weak pulses are not very specific and are often due to hypothermia, centralization from shock, and catecholamine or opioid medication.
c) **False.** Determination of the ABI is also crucial in the evaluation of acute traumatic vascular injury and can be applied quickly and reliably. A drop in ABI to < 0.9 and especially differences between sides can be a strong indication of an arterial lesion. Especially in combination with clinical signs of peripheral ischemia, the ABI has a sensitivity and specificity of $> 90\%$. However, this does not confirm a vascular lesion. Often, a hematoma or bone fragment can cause external compression of the arteries, leading to a pulse deficit or a drop in ABI, without an arterial wall lesion or arterial occlusion being present.
d) **False.** Even an initially unremarkable pulse status and a normal ABI in an injured limb do not rule out limb ischemia over time. There are several reasons for this:
   I. The initial examination finding was incorrect and an arterial lesion is missed.
   II. There is an intimal lesion without hemodynamic relevance (so foot pulses are correctly documented as strong), but an arterial thrombosis with subsequent ischemia develops over time.
   III. An expanding hematoma compresses the artery, but this rarely leads to ischemia.

IV. A manifest traumatic compartment syndrome leads to ischemia due to the compartment pressure rising above systolic blood pressure. Especially in closed tibial shaft and forearm fractures, compartment syndrome develops in 3–5% of cases, which clinically, in addition to soft tissue swelling and tension, initially manifests as ischemic symptoms.

Therefore, further monitoring of peripheral perfusion, motor function, and sensation in limb injuries, especially tibial and forearm fractures, is essential and must be documented accordingly.

e) **Correct.** Constrictive dressings above or at the level of soft tissue and/or bone injury can both hinder assessment of the extent of soft tissue injury and distort the pulse status obtained. Therefore, as the initial examiner, one should always ensure optimal examination conditions and avoid sources of error. Even with the now widespread and widely available polytrauma CT scans, the importance of physical examination should not be underestimated and must be continually practiced.

Question

13. Which statements about traumatic aortic rupture are correct?

a) Aortic rupture is a rare injury of the thoracic aorta caused by high-velocity trauma or massive impact/deceleration trauma.
b) It is most often observed in atherosclerotically pre-damaged vessels.
c) It is classified into 4 types.
d) The treatment of choice is open aortic replacement.
e) The site at the transition from the aortic arch to the descending aorta is also referred to as the “loco typico.”

Answers

a) **Correct.** In aortic rupture, there is a tear in the aortic wall at the transition from the mobile aortic arch to the fixed descending aorta, usually due to high-speed trauma.
b) **False.** It often occurs in young people (m > f) with otherwise healthy vessels. The pathomechanism is abrupt deceleration at high speed, in which the mobile part of the thoracic aorta (aortic arch) is thrown forward and torn from the fixed part of the descending aorta.
c) **Correct.** Traumatic aortic rupture is classified according to the extent of bleeding complications into type 1 (no bleeding, isolated intimal injury),

type 2 (intramural hematoma, no extravascular bleeding), type 3 (contained rupture), and type 4 (free rupture).

d) **False.** The treatment of choice is endovascular repair using TEVAR (thoracic endovascular aortic repair). The open approach was used until the introduction of endovascular techniques and was associated with extremely high mortality.

e) **Correct.** This is also referred to as traumatic aortic rupture at the "loco typico," also known as the aortic isthmus. This is a vulnerable region of the aorta directly after the origin of the left subclavian artery and the obliterated ductus arteriosus botalli.

Aorta

12

Question

1. Which statements about acute aortic syndrome are correct?

a) Acute aortic syndrome (AAS) refers to three potentially life-threatening conditions: acute dissection, intramural hematoma (IMH), and penetrating aortic ulcer (PAU).
b) Acute aortic dissection is the most common form of acute aortic syndrome, accounting for 70–80% of cases.
c) Acute aortic syndrome is rarely missed due to its clear symptomatology.
d) Syphilis was once a common cause of aortic diseases.
e) The morphological difference between intramural hematoma and aortic dissection is that the intima remains intact in the case of a hematoma.

Answers

a) **Correct.** Along with acute coronary syndrome and pulmonary embolism, AAS is one of the most important differential diagnoses of chest pain. The mortality rate is very high, at around 80%.
b) **Correct.** Acute aortic dissection was first described in 1760 by Dr. Nicholis, the personal physician to King George II, and has since been recognized as a distinct disease entity. It accounts for about 80% of AAS cases, with an incidence of 2–4/100,000/year in Central Europe. IMH and PAU each account for 10% of AAS cases and were discovered significantly later. Theodore Shennan (a surgeon from Edinburgh, 1869–1948) first described PAU in 1934. IMH was long considered a special form of acute dissection.

S. Regus, *Vascular Surgery: Questions and Answers*,
https://doi.org/10.1007/978-3-662-73387-5_12

c) **Incorrect.** AAS is missed in one out of four patients. Common differential diagnoses include acute coronary syndrome, pulmonary embolism, and stroke. For this reason, it is important to consider the diagnosis of AAS in cases of acute chest pain and, if necessary, to initiate further diagnostics using CTA. In addition to taking a medical history (family history, genetic disorders such as Marfan, Ehlers-Danlos, and Loeys-Dietz syndromes), elevated D-dimers can be an important indicator of aortic pathology.
d) **Correct.** Before the antibiotic era, aortic changes due to syphilis were relatively common. Histologically, this leads to loosening of the vessel wall, especially the elastic fibers, with subsequent dilation due to loss of elasticity. With the introduction of antibiotic therapy, this disease pattern is now rarely seen.
e) **Correct.** In intramural hematoma, which is sometimes considered a precursor to dissection, there is bleeding into the media due to rupture of the vasa vasorum, while the intima remains intact. IMH can occur throughout the aorta, but is most commonly seen in the thoracic aorta. Here, similar to the classification of dissection, it can also be divided into Stanford type A and B pathologies.

Question

2. Which statements about aortic dissection are correct?

a) In aortic dissection, there is typically a tear in the intima and formation of a second vascular lumen.
b) Classification is according to De Bakey or Stanford.
c) The abdominal aorta is most commonly affected.
d) The most common complication is rupture, followed by coronary, cerebral, or viscerorenal malperfusion.
e) The mortality rate of conservatively treated Stanford type A dissection is 95%.

Answers

a) **Correct.** Especially arteries with pre-existing atherosclerotic damage and genetic disorders (Marfan syndrome, Ehlers-Danlos syndrome, Loeys-Dietz syndrome) are associated with an increased risk of dissection.
b) **Correct.** The De Bakey classification is divided into I, II, and III.
   I= Aorta ascendens, distal extension variable
   II= limited to the ascending aorta
   III= Aorta descendens (the boundary is the left subclavian artery)

The Stanford classification is divided into A and B
A= Aorta ascendens, distal extension variable (80%).
B = Aorta descendens (boundary is the left subclavian artery, 20%)
The Stanford classification is more commonly used in clinical practice; the difference from the De Bakey classification is merely the absence of a separate category for dissection limited to the ascending aorta.

c) **Incorrect.** The abdominal aorta is affected in only 5–10% of cases, whereas the thoracic aorta is the main site of manifestation. The ascending aorta is most commonly affected, accounting for 60–70% of all cases, followed by the descending aorta with 10–20%, and the aortic arch with 5–10% involvement.
d) **Incorrect.** The most common complication in Stanford type A dissection is aortic valve insufficiency (70–80%) with shock symptoms and dyspnea. Other common complications include occlusion of major aortic branches. The most prominent are cerebral, coronary, or spinal malperfusion, which occur in up to 50–70% of cases. Cerebral ischemia or embolization is most common (5–13%), followed by myocardial infarction (about 2–9%) and spinal cord ischemia (0.5–5%).
e) **Incorrect.** The mortality rate for conservatively treated type A dissections is 50–75%, and about 20% with surgery. Interestingly, despite the severity of the disease, about 25–50% of conservatively treated patients with type A dissection survive. A dissection is considered chronic if the thoracic pain event occurred > 14 days ago.

Question

3. Which statements about intramural hematoma (IMH) and penetrating aortic ulcer (PAU) are correct?

a) PAU most commonly occurs in the abdominal aorta.
b) PAU has a high rupture rate and should always be treated.
c) IMH can progress to a dissection.
d) For a PAU, a landing zone of 1 cm in healthy aorta is sufficient.
e) Patients with connective tissue disorders very often have a PAU as a precursor to dissection.

Answers

a) **Incorrect.** PAU affects the thoracic aorta in > ¾ of cases, most commonly the descending aorta.

b) **Incorrect.** Not every PAU requires treatment upon diagnosis. A distinction is made between complicated and uncomplicated penetrating aortic ulcers, with the latter generally managed conservatively. Complicated means
   I. Presence of recurrent pain or
   II. Initial diameter > 20 mm or
   III. Depth > 10 mm or
   IV. Progression of the total aortic diameter.

   However, the location of the PAU also plays a role. PAUs of the ascending aorta have a relatively high risk of complications, with a rupture rate of up to 60%. Dissections according to Stanford A occur at a similar rate and always require emergency treatment. The risk of rupture or dissection of a PAU in the descending (5–10%) or abdominal aorta (2–3%) is much lower.
c) **Correct.** IMH can develop into acute dissection if there is a complete separation of the vessel wall layers. This is not yet the case in IMH. The risk of complete separation and development of acute aortic dissection from an IMH is greatest in the first 3 days. Therefore, IMH should be closely monitored in an intensive care setting upon diagnosis, with strict and frequent controls. In particular, hypertensive crises must be prevented. A CT scan is recommended after 24–48 hours.
d) **Incorrect.** For PAU, a sufficiently long prosthesis should also be selected to ensure adequate sealing. A 10 cm long prosthesis is often sufficient, sometimes a 15 cm one. The proximal and distal landing zones should each be at least 3 cm long.
e) **Incorrect.** Patients with connective tissue disorders (Marfan, Ehlers-Danlos, and Loeys-Dietz syndromes) rarely have a PAU, but primarily dissections or dissecting aneurysms, and sometimes an IMH. These aortic wall changes are manifestations of the connective tissue disorder and weakness. PAU, on the other hand, arises in the vast majority of cases due to atherosclerosis, which patients with congenital aortic syndromes rarely have. Therefore, PAU is a typical (albeit rare) cause of acute aortic syndrome in patients with a cardiovascular risk profile. The aortic wall in the area of the PAU or along its entire length is massively calcified. If these calcifications are absent, acquired (e.g., traumatic or iatrogenic aortic injuries) or infection-related lesions are highly suspected. Especially in cases of suspected bacterial contamination, the indication for endovascular treatment should be critically reviewed and, if at all, considered only as a bridging solution, e.g., in the event of acute bleeding complications. Ideally, open reconstruction with autologous or xenogeneic replacement material should be performed.

Question

4. Which statements about thoracoabdominal aortic aneurysm (TAAA) are correct?

a) 20% of all patients with an aortic aneurysm have a thoracoabdominal aneurysm.
b) Thoracoabdominal aneurysms are classified according to Crawford into types I–VI.
c) Typical symptoms of a TAAA are retrosternal, lumbar, or abdominal pain, shortness of breath, and hoarseness.
d) Horner's syndrome is another, very rare clinical sign of TAAA.
e) In the differential diagnosis, thoracic aortic aneurysm should also be considered in cases of shortness of breath, stridor, and superior vena cava syndrome.

Answers

a) **Incorrect.** Thoracoabdominal aneurysms account for < 3% of all aortic aneurysms. Of abdominal aneurysms, 95% are infrarenal, only 5% are juxta- or suprarenal. When considering thoracic aneurysms alone, about 30% extend below the diaphragm.
b) **Incorrect.** Classification is indeed according to Crawford, but into types I–IV. In types I and II, the aneurysm begins at the level of the left subclavian artery; in type I, the distal extension is up to above the renal arteries, and any extension below the renal arteries is classified as type II. In type III, the aneurysm begins along the descending aorta, and in type IV at the level of the diaphragm.
c) **Correct.** These symptoms can be explained by compression as the aneurysm increases in size, and hoarseness occurs when the recurrent laryngeal nerve is affected.
d) **Correct.** Horner's syndrome in TAAA can be explained by compression of the cervical sympathetic trunk, particularly the superior cervical ganglion. However, there are fewer than 10 case reports in the literature of Horner's syndrome caused by compression from a thoracoabdominal aortic aneurysm.
e) **Correct.** Compression of the trachea can cause shortness of breath and stridor; compression of the superior vena cava (SVC) can additionally cause swelling in the neck and upper extremity. Other differential diagnoses include decompensated heart failure, acute myocardial infarction with right heart failure, pneumonia, and pulmonary embolism.

Question

5. Which statements about the CERAB procedure are correct?

a) The CERAB procedure is an endovascular repair for aortoiliac stenoses.
b) The results after CERAB are better than after open surgical therapy.
c) The so-called BeGraft® stent graft is often used.
d) Unlike the kissing stent technique, the CERAB procedure must be performed under general anesthesia with intubation.
e) The development of the CERAB procedure is based on the results of the COBEST trial.

Answers

a) **Correct.** CERAB stands for **C**overed **e**ndovascular **r**epair of **a**ortic **b**ifurcation. This is an endovascular variant of the kissing stent technique for aortoiliac stenoses or occlusions. In contrast to the kissing stent technique, covered stents or stent grafts are used and deployed both aortically and bilaterally in the iliac arteries.
b) **Correct.** The BeGraft® stent graft from Bentley InnoMed (Hechingen, Germany) is frequently used for the CERAB procedure. These are aortic and peripheral stent grafts covered with ePTFE. The available aortic diameters range from 12–24 mm with lengths of 19–59 mm. For the iliac extensions, prostheses with diameters of 5–10 mm and lengths up to 58 mm are available.
c) **Incorrect.** In most cases, the CERAB procedure can be performed under local anesthesia, which is a major advantage given the often pronounced multimorbidity of these patients.
d) **Incorrect.** The 5-year patency rates after open surgical therapy for aortoiliac TASC C and D lesions are still better than after the CERAB procedure. However, the results after CERAB are better than after the uncovered kissing stent technique.
e) **Correct.** In the COBEST trial (Covered Versus Balloon Expandable Stent), a randomized multicenter study published in 2011, results after covered stent implantation were compared for the first time with those of uncovered stents, both using the kissing technique. Patency rates for TASC B lesions were comparable, but covered stents showed better results for TASC C and D lesions. This subsequently led to the idea of extending with a covered prosthesis aortically, from which the CERAB procedure was developed.

The basic idea was to achieve better aortoiliac geometry through additional aortic stent implantation and to reduce intimal hyperplasia and embolization by using covered stents.

Question

6. Which statements about mid-aortic syndrome are correct?

a) Mid-aortic syndrome is a disease of advanced age.
b) Typical symptoms of mid-aortic syndrome include elevated blood pressure in the upper extremities.
c) Claudication symptoms are reported only in exceptional cases in mid-aortic syndrome.
d) The treatment of choice for mid-aortic syndrome is interventional therapy using bioresorbable stents (vascular scaffolds).
e) The primary surgical procedures are TEA with patch plasty and, if necessary, reimplantation of the visceral arteries.

Answers

a) **Incorrect.** Mid-aortic syndrome is a congenital disease that typically manifests in childhood or adolescence. It is a narrowing or complete obliteration of the abdominal aorta in the visceral artery segment (section 4).
b) **Correct.** The most commonly first detected symptom is arterial hypertension, which is often therapy-resistant. This is often accompanied by headaches, dizziness, and epistaxis. The arterial hypertension is caused on the one hand by increased resistance due to the aortic stenosis and the resulting volume overload of the structures above. Another cause is impaired renal perfusion and the resulting renovascular hypertension, which is triggered by activation of the renin-angiotensin cascade.
c) **Incorrect.** The most common symptom leading to diagnosis is claudication or weakness and loss of performance in the lower extremity. Parents describe their children as "reluctant to walk." The serious renovascular hypertension, which is also present in most cases, is often recognized too late. This is because it causes no or only atypical symptoms in the early stages. Only in advanced stages and when complications or organ damage occur is further diagnostic workup initiated.
d) **Incorrect.** In principle, both interventional and surgical therapy are possible. Intensive research is underway to develop bioresorbable stents for use

in the aorta in children, but currently none of the promising materials and products are approved. When conventional stents or stent grafts are used, restenosis often occurs after completion of physical growth, so sometimes the growth phase is awaited before interventional therapy. However, if there is severe or uncontrolled arterial hypertension, a wait-and-see approach is contraindicated.

e) **Correct.** TEA with patch plasty should be preferred if possible. Xenogeneic material, usually bovine pericardium, is recommended as patch material. A tube can also be formed from the latter and used as a replacement. In addition, reimplantation of the renal and visceral arteries is usually necessary. If medically justifiable, surgery should be performed after completion of growth to avoid restenosis.

Question

7. Which statements about coarctation of the aorta are correct?

a) Another term for coarctation of the aorta is aortic isthmus stenosis.
b) Aortic isthmus stenosis is classified into pre-, juxta-, and postductal forms.
c) The preductal form of aortic isthmus stenosis usually manifests in early adulthood.
d) Coarctatio literally means narrowing, constriction, or crowding together.
e) The most important immediate measure in the preductal form is a prostaglandin E1 infusion to keep the ductus arteriosus open.

Answers

a) **Correct.** Coarctation of the aorta is a stenosis of the aortic isthmus and is one of the very rare congenital aortic diseases. Anatomically, the aortic isthmus is located between the left subclavian artery and the origin of the first pair of intercostal arteries. In this section of the aorta, the ductus arteriosus Botalli is also usually found.

b) **Correct.** The classification in relation to the ductus is clinically significant because, especially in the preductal form, there is usually an urgent, sometimes even emergency, indication for surgery.

c) **Correct.** The preductal form is the most dangerous type, as it often leads to massive left heart strain and decompensation shortly after birth, and the infant's life can only be saved by emergency cardiac surgery. The postductal form is often not diagnosed until adulthood and is also significantly rarer than the preductal form. Pathophysiologically, the decisive factor for the life-threatening nature of the preductal form is that there is no collateralization from the preductal to the postductal aorta, since the preductal aorta is virtually not perfused during the embryonic stage. No oxygenation takes place in the lungs; oxygen-rich blood comes via the inferior vena cava from the umbilical vein. After birth, gas exchange must occur in the lungs, and consequently, perfusion of the preductal aorta becomes vital, which can lead to massive overload and decompensation of the left ventricle. In the postductal form, collaterals must already be established and developed during the embryonic stage to ensure perfusion of the lower extremities. As a result, there is no significant pressure load on the left ventricle.

d) **Correct.** Coarctatio comes from Latin and literally means to contract, to connect, to crowd together. Since the aorta can be narrowed at any point, coarctation of the abdominal aorta in the visceral artery segment can also be referred to as abdominal coarctation. However, the term mid-aortic syndrome has become established here, which is also internationally accepted.
e) **Correct.** Alprostadil (also known as prostaglandin E1) leads to vasodilation and can be administered as an infusion therapy in early infancy to keep the ductus Botalli open. This infusion can be life-saving until surgical intervention is performed.

13 Visceral Vascular Diseases

Question

1. Which statements about visceral artery aneurysms (VAA) are correct?

a) The indication for invasive exclusion of an asymptomatic aneurysm exists from a diameter of 2 cm.
b) Symptomatic aneurysms should be excluded regardless of diameter.
c) Ruptured aneurysms have a similarly high mortality as contained ruptured abdominal aortic aneurysms.
d) The cause of VAA is usually atherosclerosis.
e) True aneurysms diagnosed during pregnancy should be excluded upon diagnosis, regardless of diameter.

Answers

a) **Correct.** Additionally, in the case of size progression of > 0.5 cm/year or if the diameter is three times larger than the adjacent normal diameter.
b) **Correct.** If abdominal pain is attributable to the aneurysm, the indication for exclusion should be made upon diagnosis.
c) **Incorrect.** Since VAAs usually rupture freely, and not in a contained manner, the mortality is higher than with aortic rupture and is > 80%.
d) **Correct.** Another important cause is fibromuscular dysplasia, especially in younger patients.
e) **Correct.** In principle, exclusion should be performed in women of childbearing age regardless of diameter, as the risk of rupture is significantly increased during pregnancy and poses a danger to both mother and unborn child.

S. Regus, *Vascular Surgery: Questions and Answers*,
https://doi.org/10.1007/978-3-662-73387-5_13

Question

2. Which statements about abdominal angina (AA) are correct?

a) AA typically presents with postprandial pain that disappears 2–3 hours after food intake.
b) In AA, typically only one of the three mesenteric vessels (CA, SMA, IMA) is stenosed or occluded.
c) AA is a common disease of advanced age.
d) Abdominal hyperperfusion syndrome is a rare complication after revascularization of stenosed visceral arteries.
e) Surgical reconstruction is usually performed as an aortomesenteric bypass, preferably using the GSV as bypass material.

Answers

a) **Correct.** The classic clinical symptomatology consists of diffuse abdominal pain and sometimes postprandial diarrhea, which disappears 2–3 hours after food intake. In addition, patients often report a chronically increasing symptomatology and weight loss.
b) **Incorrect.** In AA, at least 2 of the 3 mesenteric arteries are typically stenosed or occluded. This is due to the usually pronounced collateralization between the supply territories. Even if the SMA is occluded, patients with normal IMA and CA are usually asymptomatic, and stenoses or occlusions seen on imaging are merely incidental findings.
c) **Incorrect.** AA is a rare disease with a prevalence of 0.03%. It predominantly affects people of advanced age; in young patients, it is extremely rare and is either associated with genetic syndromes or excessive nicotine abuse. Interestingly, the prevalence of asymptomatic stenoses of the visceral arteries is much higher, up to 30%.
d) **Correct.** There are rare case reports of hyperperfusion syndromes after successful revascularization of stenosed or occluded visceral arteries. For example, there are case reports of splenic ruptures after stent PTA of the celiac trunk and mesenteric arteries, subsequently requiring emergency splenectomy. However, these are extremely rare complications; overall, interventional therapy of AA carries a low mortality risk.
e) **Incorrect.** In most cases, the common iliac artery is chosen as the donor vessel, as this avoids the need for cross-clamping the aorta. The latter is associated with a significant burden for the usually multimorbid patient

population. Synthetic grafts have become established as bypass material, showing comparable results to autologous materials (especially the GSV). No difference was found between polyester and PTFE, so the choice is left to the surgeon. Ring-reinforced prostheses with a diameter of 6–8 mm are recommended. The so-called "lazy C" configuration has become established for intra-abdominal retrograde bypass routing to avoid kinking stenoses and immediate occlusions. It does not matter whether the right or left common iliac artery is chosen as the donor vessel.

Question

3. Which statements about acute mesenteric infarction are correct?

a) The clinical symptomatology of acute mesenteric infarction is clear and easy to diagnose.
b) The typical patient with acute mesenteric infarction is of advanced age, multimorbid, and suffers from cardiac arrhythmias.
c) Most often, the cause of acute mesenteric infarction is an arterial embolism, rarely an arterial thrombosis.
d) If a proximal, 2 cm long arterial thrombosis of the SMA is detected in the presence of an underlying stenosis and typical clinical symptoms of mesenteric infarction, laparotomy should in principle be performed first, followed by interventional therapy with stent PTA.
e) Laboratory determination of lactate is an indispensable component in the suspected diagnosis of mesenteric ischemia and should in principle be determined in all types of abdominal pain.

Answers

a) **Incorrect.** Correct diagnosis of mesenteric infarction is challenging. Mesenteric ischemia is often not initially recognized correctly because the symptoms are nonspecific. However, due to the ischemic tolerance of only a few hours, this diagnostic delay often has fatal consequences for the patient. It is not uncommon for bowel ischemia to be recognized too late, and the subsequent laparotomy must be terminated prematurely. In these cases, intraoperatively, a completely black small intestine is typically seen, making reconstruction and resection no longer promising. Thus, the mortality of acute mesenteric infarction remains 60–80%, despite the now widely available CT diagnostics.
b) **Correct.** Typically, patients with mesenteric infarction are elderly (usually over 70 years old) with corresponding cardiovascular risk factors. Atrial

fibrillation is often known or newly diagnosed. They are usually in a very poor general condition and are seriously ill.

c) **Correct.** Of the four causes of acute mesenteric circulatory disorders—arterial embolism (50%), arterial thrombosis (25%), non-occlusive disease NOMI (15%), and venous thrombosis (10%)—embolism is the most common, accounting for about half of cases. In the vast majority (85%) of cases of acute ischemia, the SMA is affected. As with limb ischemia, in visceral ischemia, clinical symptoms are mild if there is good collateralization with chronically progressive stenosis.
d) **Incorrect.** If the patient is stable and CT does not already suggest advanced bowel wall damage (pneumatosis), revascularization should be performed as quickly as possible. In the case of short-segment proximal stenoses, interventional therapy with stent PTA has proven effective, followed immediately by surgery. The reverse approach—first laparotomy, then intervention—is also possible, but this more often leads to delayed reperfusion and a significantly increased risk of anastomotic insufficiency. Of course, laparotomy can also be combined with surgical mesenteric reconstruction, but this involves a much longer operative time and increases the mortality risk in these usually elderly, multimorbid patients.
e) **Incorrect.** Lactate is, on the one hand, a nonspecific laboratory parameter and, especially in the early stage of mesenteric ischemia, is of little use. Often, a significantly elevated lactate level is only measurable in the late stage. However, elevated lactate levels in the early stage are also not proof of mesenteric infarction, although the sensitivity is relatively high at almost 90%. In many hospitals, lactate determination is routinely included in serological testing in both the emergency department and intensive care unit for patients with mesenteric circulatory disorders. However, the specificity of lactate diagnostics is low, at less than 50%. It is also worth mentioning the determination of D-dimers. These also have low specificity. However, in daily practice, it has been shown that especially in the early stage, negative D-dimers also have a very high diagnostic value, as the probability of mesenteric infarction with negative D-dimers is very low. The same applies to normal lactate levels.

   In summary, the following practical benefit can be established for clinical routine: Negative D-dimers and normal lactate levels virtually rule out mesenteric ischemia. This is due to the high negative predictive value of both parameters.

Question

4. Which statements about non-occlusive mesenteric ischemia are correct?

a) So-called NOMI (non-occlusive mesenteric ischemia) is a visceral circulatory disorder in which the mesenteric vessels show no stenoses.
b) Non-occlusive mesenteric ischemia (NOMI) is as common as the occlusive form.
c) There are no therapeutic measures other than circulatory stabilization.
d) Women are significantly more frequently affected.
e) There are evidence-based diagnostic and therapeutic recommendations.

Answers

a) **Correct.** In NOMI, there are no stenoses of the mesenteric vessels. The causes are rather severe comorbidities, a cardiovascular procedure with circulatory dysfunction, acute myocardial infarction, or post-resuscitation. These lead to a visceral perfusion disorder.
b) **Incorrect.** NOMI is less common than the occlusive form, but with about 20–30% of cases, it is still not rare. However, the mortality is > 90%, which is mostly due to the underlying diseases.
c) **Incorrect.** If the patient's condition allows, exploratory laparotomy should be performed, and if the suspected diagnosis is confirmed, intra-arterial administration of vasodilators (papaverine) should be started.
d) **Incorrect.** No gender-specific differences are known. The prevalence of NOMI increases with age and number of comorbidities.
e) **Incorrect.** Due to the rarity of the disease, there is little scientific literature, and only in the form of case reports or series. The available evidence is currently limited to expert opinions.

Question

5. Which statements about the anatomy of the mesenteric vessels are correct?

a) The celiac trunk, superior mesenteric artery, and inferior mesenteric artery are important mesenteric vessels.
b) The supplied tissue sections are always end-arterial territories.

c) Branches of the celiac trunk are the common hepatic artery, splenic artery, and left gastric artery.
d) Reconstruction of the celiac trunk, e.g., in an emergency due to a bleeding complication, is essential to prevent ischemia.
e) Simple ligation of the portal vein is usually well tolerated.

Answers

a) **Correct.** These three branches from the abdominal aorta are responsible for the arterial supply of the entire gastrointestinal tract.
b) **Incorrect.** There are collaterals, the most important being the Riolan anastomosis between the superior and inferior mesenteric arteries.
c) **Correct.** These are the most important branches. Thus, the celiac trunk and its branches supply the liver, spleen, stomach, and esophagus.
d) **Incorrect.** There are case reports of successful ligation of the celiac trunk, usually in the context of aneurysm rupture, without postoperative ischemic symptoms in the liver, stomach, or esophagus. However, it is important to check for a strong backflow from the peripheral vessel segment, which indicates good collateralization.
e) **Correct.** Especially in traumatic injuries of the portal vein and compromised patient physiology, complex reconstruction is contraindicated. However, a second-look operation should be aimed for. In the case of simultaneous injury to the hepatic artery, the portal vein must definitely be reconstructed.

Question

6. Which statements about renal artery stenoses are correct?

a) High-grade renal artery stenoses, even if diagnosed incidentally, should always be treated invasively.
b) The most common cause of renal artery stenoses is atherosclerosis, followed by fibromuscular dysplasia (FMD).
c) The most common clinical sign of renal artery stenosis is arterial hypertension.
d) For interventional therapy, balloon angioplasty alone is usually sufficient.
e) A clinically asymptomatic unilateral renal artery stenosis should always be treated during an EVAR procedure.

Answers

a) **Incorrect.** Renal artery stenoses are often discovered incidentally, frequently during CT diagnostics for clarification of abdominal pain or a vascular disease (aneurysms, PAD). The indication for invasive therapy should be made critically due to the peri-interventional complication risk. Indications would be medically uncontrollable arterial hypertension, otherwise unexplained renal insufficiency with rising retention parameters (especially in diabetics), as well as younger patients with high-grade stenoses to prevent acute renal artery occlusion.
b) **Correct.** In about 90%, the cause of renal artery stenoses is atherosclerosis. Other causes are FMD with about 10% and very rarely (< 1%) other causes such as tumor compression or vasculitis. FMD is observed much more frequently in women than in men, especially in younger women in the 3rd–4th decade of life. If men have FMD, they are usually older.
c) **Correct.** Arterial hypertension is the most common clinical sign of renal artery stenosis, followed by renal insufficiency with rising retention parameters and reduction of glomerular filtration rate. However, other causes of renal dysfunction should definitely be excluded. The prevalence of renal artery stenoses among hypertensive patients is 1–5% and thus very rare. The cause of arterial hypertension is activation of renin production, which increases renin-angiotensin-aldosterone synthesis. Since activation of renin production only occurs with stenoses of 80% or more, clinically asymptomatic renal artery stenoses are much more frequently diagnosed as incidental findings in CT angiography.
d) **Incorrect.** Balloon angioplasty alone often leads to recurrent stenoses or so-called recoil directly during the intervention, so primary stent implantation is generally recommended. In young patients with short-segment FMD-induced stenosis, balloon angioplasty alone should still be attempted initially. Short (9–20 mm) bare metal stents with a diameter of 5–6 millimeters are used. For ostial stenoses, these stents should protrude 1–2 mm into the aorta and be dilated accordingly to reduce the risk of ostial restenosis.
e) **Incorrect.** Although there is no evidence from larger studies, as renal artery stenosis is a rare disease, there is also no S3 guideline, but only an S2k guideline from the German Society for Vascular Surgery. Experts agreed that an asymptomatic unilateral renal artery stenosis should not be treated during an infrarenal endovascular aortic procedure (EVAR), as the complication risk likely far outweighs any potential benefit for the patient.

Question

7. Which statements about the surgical therapy of visceral vascular diseases are correct?

a) The treatment of visceral artery stenoses is a domain of open vascular surgery.
b) The aorta should be chosen as the donor vessel for visceral bypasses.
c) In case of clinical suspicion of ischemic bowel wall damage, radiological intervention of occluded visceral arteries should be performed immediately.
d) The GSV should preferably be used for mesenteric bypasses.
e) False aneurysms of the visceral arteries are guideline-based excluded from a diameter of 2 cm.

Answers

a) **Incorrect.** Visceral artery stenoses are now mostly treated interventionally. It is important that the result of dilation is usually stabilized with a stent, otherwise the risk of recurrent stenosis is very high. Especially proximal stenoses can be technically very well treated by interventional radiologists. The further peripherally the intervention is performed, the greater the risk of complications and recurrences. As with the treatment of arterial stenoses in the extremities, longer-segment stenoses or occlusions, depending on the general condition and operability of the patient, should primarily be approached surgically.
b) **Incorrect.** The common iliac artery, less commonly the external iliac artery, is usually chosen as the donor vessel for visceral bypasses. The abdominal aorta is used less frequently, e.g., for short interpositions or reimplantations. Advantages of the iliac vessels as donor vessels are that the cardiopulmonary intra- and perioperative complication rate is reduced, as aortic clamping can be avoided. It is also important to route the bypass in a wide arc (lazy C configuration) to avoid tension and compression of the graft as well as intra-abdominal structures. The guiding structure for bypass routing is the ipsilateral iliac vessel and the abdominal aorta up to the original origin of the reconstructed artery.
c) **Incorrect.** If there is clinical (peritonism), laboratory (elevated lactate, D-dimer, and inflammatory markers), and radiological (air inclusions in the bowel wall) suspicion of bowel ischemia, emergency laparotomy should be

performed. Depending on the extent of ischemia and bowel wall damage, affected bowel segments must be removed and arterial perfusion restored at the same time. If more than 100 cm of small intestine must be removed, short bowel syndrome is inevitable. If less than 50 cm of small intestine remains, survival is hardly possible. In the case of a completely "black" bowel, only palliative therapy remains due to the hopeless prognosis, as the condition is not survivable.

d) **Correct.** The GSV is also considered the ideal bypass material for visceral artery reconstructions. Alternatively, a pelvic vein or synthetic material can be used. Nevertheless, it should be remembered that the GSV should be initially draped in a sterile manner to allow for easy harvesting. Synthetic material should be avoided if possible, especially due to the risk of infection. Both PTFE and polyester prostheses show good patency rates; many surgeons prefer externally reinforced prostheses.

e) **Incorrect.** A pseudoaneurysm of the visceral arteries should be excluded upon diagnosis, as the risk of rupture is incalculable and relatively high. The most common causes of false aneurysms are pancreatitis and post-laparoscopic procedures. The affected arteries are therefore mainly peripancreatic arteries such as the splenic, gastroduodenal, pancreaticoduodenal, and hepatic arteries. Treatment is usually endovascular by embolization or implantation of covered stents (so-called flow-diverter stents).

Septic Vascular Surgery 14

Question

1. Which statements regarding perioperative infection prophylaxis are correct?

a) Changing gloves intraoperatively before touching and implanting a synthetic prosthesis has been proven to reduce the risk of bypass infection.
b) Perioperative antibiotic prophylaxis leads to a significant reduction in infection rates.
c) Rifampicin-soaked prostheses have significantly fewer infections than untreated implants.
d) Shaving of the surgical site should be performed well in advance of the procedure, ideally > 24 hours beforehand.
e) Skin disinfection of the surgical area is performed immediately before sterile draping using alcohol-based solutions.

Answers

a) **False.** There is no scientific evidence supporting the effectiveness of glove changes in preventing bypass infections. However, the available studies are limited, consisting of isolated single-center studies.
b) **True.** According to current studies, perioperative antibiotic prophylaxis is the most important and effective measure against wound infections and septic prosthesis complications in surgical medicine. However, perioperative antibiotic administration for longer than 24 hours offers no advantage

S. Regus, *Vascular Surgery: Questions and Answers*,
https://doi.org/10.1007/978-3-662-73387-5_14

compared to administration for less than 24 hours. This applies to both wound and prosthesis infections.

c) **False.** Rifampicin-soaked prostheses do not have a lower infection rate than unsoaked prostheses. In the few available studies comparing rifampicin-soaked prostheses with untreated implants, no significant difference in the number of prosthesis infections was found. However, there was a certain trend toward infection reduction. Nevertheless, the results were not significant, so further studies with larger case numbers may be awaited.
d) **False.** Shaving of the surgical site should indeed be performed outside the operating area, but as close as possible to the time of surgery. In many hospitals, it has proven effective to perform shaving shortly before the patient is called from the ward. Since the use of disposable razors has even led to an increase in wound infections in studies, only electric razors are now recommended. Disposable razors, which are still often found in operating rooms, should be consistently removed and no longer used for shaving the surgical site.
e) **True.** Skin disinfection is performed in the operating room immediately before draping, either by the already sterilely dressed OR nurse or by the surgical assistants or the surgeon themselves. Even though the terms are often used interchangeably, there is a difference between antiseptics and disinfectants: antiseptics are applied to the skin, while disinfectants are used for treating inanimate surfaces. The goal of both measures and solutions is to reduce the microbial density of the respective surface. In the operating room, an alcohol-based colored antiseptic (e.g., Cutasept G®) is usually used, which has a contact time of 2 minutes. The procedure is generally repeated three times, either by wiping with solution-soaked swabs or by spraying. For small and clearly defined surgical areas, colorless solutions (e.g., Cutasept F®) can also be used. G stands for colored and F for colorless.

Question

2. Which statements regarding septic vascular complications are correct?

a) Typical pathogens of septic erosion hemorrhages are gram-negative bacteria.
b) A septic erosion hemorrhage in shunt surgery is more common in lower arm than in upper arm shunts.

c) Every hypoechoic rim around a peripheral bypass must be aspirated and the aspirate examined bacteriologically.
d) In cases of infected groin, the so-called obturator bypass is a common reconstruction option.
e) Xenogeneic transplants are a promising alternative for vascular reconstruction in septic bypass surgery.

Answers

a) **False.** Most often, these are gram-positive pathogens, predominantly Staphylococcus, Streptococcus, and Enterococcus species. Staphylococcus epidermidis is one of the most important nosocomial pathogens. Among the gram-negative pathogens, E. coli and Pseudomonas should be mentioned. Over the past decades, infections with staphylococci have decreased, whereas pathogens such as Klebsiella, Pseudomonas, and E. coli have tended to increase.
b) **False.** Overall, septic erosion hemorrhage is very rare; however, due to the regular punctures, especially with synthetic shunts, it is a serious complication. It occurs in about 3–5% of shunt patients. The brachial artery is more frequently affected than the radial artery; in emergencies, the supplying vessel can be ligated. Studies have shown that the risk of upper limb loss after emergency ligation of the brachial artery is low.
c) **False.** It is not uncommon to see a hypoechoic rim around peripheral bypasses, especially with alloplastic materials, on ultrasound. If there are also systemic and especially local signs of inflammation (skin redness along the bypass, swelling, tenderness), the likelihood of a bypass infection is high, and an aspirate should be obtained and examined bacteriologically. Without signs of inflammation, it is most likely a differential diagnosis of an aseptic, sterile perigraft reaction. This can also be observed years after implantation. Bypass explantation should be strictly avoided.
d) **True.** The obturator bypass is an option to bypass an infected situation in the groin. Here, the bypass is anastomosed proximally to the iliac artery and then passed through the obturator foramen. The bypass runs extra-anatomically along the medial thigh and is anastomosed to the superficial femoral or popliteal artery. The disadvantage is the reduced patency rate of only 70% after 1 year and 50% after 5 years. This is most likely due to the extra-anatomic course of the bypass. However, the limb salvage rate is satisfactory at 75% after 5 years.

e) **True.** Xenogeneic materials have increasingly been used in recent years as a good alternative for vascular reconstruction in infected areas. Notably, bovine patches made from porcine pericardium should be mentioned. These have been used in cardiac surgery for some time, among other reasons due to their stable and easily suturable properties. They are also being used more frequently in vascular surgery, where previously only silver-impregnated polyester prostheses and homografts were available. Some authors report very good short- and long-term results using self-made xenogeneic tube prostheses of various diameters for anatomical reconstruction of infected areas. These biological patches are available in sizes from 1×6 cm to 10×16 cm, for example from LeMaitre (XenoSure® Biological surgical patches).

Question

3. Which statements regarding risk factors for septic vascular complications are correct?

a) The risk of a bypass infection (alloplastic) is greatest in the groin area.
b) The duration of the operation has no influence on the risk of infection.
c) Alloplastic implants that rapidly integrate into tissue are rarely infected.
d) Polyester (Dacron®) has fewer infections than PTFE due to its rougher surface.
e) Underweight is not a risk factor for vascular prosthesis infections.

Answers

a) **True.** The risk of a bypass infection is highest in the groin area, at about 6%, whereas the risk in the aorta is about 3%. Infections in the neck area or upper extremity are rare, which is why no advantage of xenogeneic replacement materials has been demonstrated for carotid bifurcation reconstructions. In the groin area, however, xenogeneic or autologous patches are preferable. The great saphenous vein (GSV) should not be used uncritically as a patch, as it would then no longer be available for a potentially necessary femoropopliteal or -crural reconstruction. In profundaplasty with an occluded SFA, the latter can be thrombendarterectomized and used as a patch.

b) **False.** The duration of the surgical procedure has been shown in four large multicenter studies[1,2,3,4] with > 60,000 included patients to have a significant impact on wound and bypass infection rates. In lower extremity surgical revascularizations lasting more than 4 hours, 40% more infections occurred than in shorter procedures. Some bias cannot be ruled out, especially since the length of the procedure may correlate with complexity and the number of previous operations, thus leading to a higher rate of infections.

c) **True.** Prostheses that are well integrated and incorporated into tissue have a lower risk of infection than non-incorporated bypasses. The faster the incorporation process occurs and is completed, the lower the risk of bacterial colonization. For this reason, for example, the treatment of alloplastic bypasses with plasma is currently the subject of intensive research. In such pretreated prostheses, a faster incorporation process has already been demonstrated in vitro and in animal experiments. This is explained by the increased surface tension that occurs after activation with cold (non-thermal) plasma.

d) **False.** According to current scientific data, there are no differences between the two most commonly used alloplastic vascular replacement materials, PTFE and polyester, in terms of tissue compatibility, infection, and early occlusion rates due to bypass thrombosis. Long-term results are also comparable, so the choice of material is left to the surgeon's personal preference.

---

[1] Aziz F, Bohr T, Lehman EB (2017) Wound disruption after lower extremity bypass surgery is a predictor of subsequent development of wound infection. Ann Vasc Surg 43:176–187.

[2] Greenblatt DY, Rajamanickam V, Mell MW (2011) Predictors of surgical site infection after open lower extremity revascularization. J Vasc Surg 54:433–439.

[3] Henke PK, Kubus J, Englesbe MJ et al (2010) A statewide consortium of surgical care: a longitudinal investigation of vascular operative procedures at 16 hospitals. Surgery 148:883–889 (discussion 889–892).

[4] Wiseman JT, Fernandes-Taylor S, Barnes ML et al. (2015) Predictors of surgical site infection after hospital discharge in patients undergoing major vascular surgery. J Vasc Surg 62:1023–1031.e1025.

e) **False.** Although scientific studies have focused on obesity and its influence on wound healing disorders and vascular prosthesis infections, and it has been shown that obesity is associated with a significantly increased risk of infection, subgroup analyses have yielded interesting findings: female gender is an independent risk factor for wound infections in the groin area, whereas a high body mass index (BMI) does not represent a risk factor here.[5] Underweight is also a risk factor for wound healing disorders and infectious complications, especially in the presence of hypoproteinemia due to malnutrition. Very thin or cachectic patients also often tend to have impaired wound healing. The development of pressure sores and decubitus ulcers along the prosthesis and in the scar area is not uncommon. Therefore, the generally important tissue-sparing preparation technique is particularly recommended in cachectic patients to avoid wound problems.

Question

4. Which statements regarding antibacterial therapy for septic complications in vascular surgery are correct?

a) Every sonographically conspicuous hypoechoic or anechoic rim around a prosthetic bypass must be treated with antibiotics, even in the absence of local or systemic signs of infection.
b) In about half of cases, the causative bacteria are gram-positive cocci.
c) Polyhexanide, octenidine dihydrochloride (OCT, Octenisept®), and povidone-iodine (PVP-iodine) can be used to irrigate infected prosthesis beds and have a bactericidal effect. Isolated cases of tissue-toxic reactions have been observed when Octenisept® was injected into very deep wounds using a syringe. This complication has been observed especially in children, so a critical or extremely cautious application is recommended in this group.
d) Sulmycin® sponges have proven very effective as a dressing on infected prosthesis beds instead of systemic antibiotic administration.
e) Cutimed®sorbact® can be applied to infected wounds and acts directly bactericidal through its components (dialkylcarbamoyl chloride = DACC).

---

[5] Arnaoutakis DJ, Scully RE, Sharma G, Shah SK, Ozaki CK, Belkin M, Nguyen LL. Impact of body mass index and gender on wound complications after lower extremity arterial surgery. J Vasc Surg. 2017 Jun;65(6):1713–1718.e1. https://doi.org/10.1016/j.jvs.2016.12.116. Epub 2017 Mar 1. PMID: 28259578.

Answers

a) **False.** In the absence of clinical or laboratory signs of infection, a randomly discovered hypoechoic rim is most likely an aseptic perigraft reaction. If all other findings are unremarkable, aspirate collection for bacteriological examination should be avoided. Otherwise, the risk of contamination and secondary prosthesis infection would be increased.
b) **False.** In over 75% of cases, the pathogens of postoperative wound infections are gram-positive bacteria, mainly staphylococci (60%) and enterococci (15%). Among gram-negative pathogens, Pseudomonas and E. coli follow, each accounting for about 10%. Other enterobacteria and fungi are very rarely detected.
c) **True.** These are antiseptics with good tissue compatibility and bactericidal effect. The recommended contact time is 5–20 minutes, which is long. Nevertheless, this should be considered and observed during intraoperative irrigation.
d) **False.** Sulmycin® (gentamicin) sponges containing gentamicin sulfate can be used locally as an adjunct in the surgical treatment of purulent inflammation of bone, bone marrow, and other infection sites. Care should be taken not to moisten the sponge, as this can cause the active ingredient to be washed out. Local allergic reactions have also been reported. The application of the sponge is an adjunctive measure and does not replace systemic antibiotic therapy.
e) **False.** Cutimed®sorbact® is a hydrophobic wound dressing that irreversibly binds bacteria and fungi without toxic local side effects. The main component is dialkylcarbamoyl chloride (DACC), which serves as a hydrophobic coating. It is a fatty acid that is hydrophobic and found in spider webs. This explains the phenomenon that water droplets adhere to spider webs without destroying or wetting them. It can therefore be applied to infected wounds and left in place for up to 7 days in some cases.

Question

5. Which statements regarding Human Acellular Vessels (HAV) are correct?

a) Human Acellular Vessels (HAV) are a biological and antigen-free vascular substitute already freely available on the market.
b) The use of HAV in shunt surgery is very promising.
c) HAV are now also used for atherosclerotic indications (PAD or CAD).

d) A disadvantage of HAV is that they cannot be stored and are therefore not readily available.
e) An advantage of HAV is the possibility of immediate puncture due to their wall thickness of > 1 mm.

Answers

a) **False.** Human Acellular Vessels (HAV) are a very promising biological vascular substitute from the company Humacyte®, but are currently still in phase 2 or 3 of clinical trials.
b) **True.** The first use of HAV in dialysis patients as part of a phase II study was initiated in 2012. Forty patients were included who received an HAV as a dialysis access. The 2-year results were very good, with no evidence of infection and no need to abandon the shunt due to complications. For this reason, follow-up was extended. Even after 5 years, no infection-related abandonment of the dialysis shunt was documented.
c) **True.** HAV are now also being used in clinical phase II and III studies for coronary artery disease and peripheral arterial occlusive disease. The results so far are very promising, and approval is likely within the next few years. The diameters of the available prostheses are currently 6 mm (for shunt and bypass surgery) and 3.5 mm for coronary reconstructions.
d) **False.** HAV are sterilely packaged and can be stored at room temperature, similar to ePTFE prostheses. They are therefore available at any time if needed.
e) **False.** Even with HAV, incorporation of the prosthesis after implantation must be awaited; as with ePTFE prostheses, 4–6 weeks are recommended. The wall thickness of the 6 mm diameter prostheses is about 0.5 mm.

Question

6. Which statements regarding homografts are correct?

a) Homografts are cryopreserved vessels from brain-dead donors.
b) Homografts are exclusively arterial vessels.
c) Cryopreserved homografts can be stored indefinitely.
d) Homografts cannot be stored in hospitals.
e) After implantation of a homograft, immunosuppression is necessary.

Answers

a) **True.** Homografts are cryopreserved and thus storable cadaveric vessels from human donors. They are therefore an allogeneic vascular substitute. Aortic vessels are preferably used.

b) **False.** There are both arterial and venous homografts. Arterial homografts are mainly used for reconstruction of central vessels, while venous homografts are primarily used in peripheral bypass surgery.

c) **False.** Homografts, even when cryopreserved, have a limited shelf life of a maximum of 5 years. This is also documented as an expiration date.

d) **False.** In principle, homografts can also be stored in hospitals, provided they have not been thawed beforehand. The storage temperature must not exceed –80 °C. In addition, the shelf life is reduced to 6 months at a storage temperature of –80 °C. Cryopreservation using liquid nitrogen achieves temperatures of < –196 °C.

e) **False.** There is no clear evidence for the benefit of immunosuppression after vascular replacement with homografts. Nevertheless, administration of cyclosporine (low-dose with serum levels of 80–110 ng/ml) and additionally a glucocorticoid (prednisolone) is recommended. This is justified by the fact that both cryopreserved and fresh homografts contain surface structures (especially the histocompatibility complex) that are involved in the rejection process.

Vascular Tumor Diseases 15

Question

1. Which statements about the epidemiology of vascular tumors are correct?

a) Vascular tumors are an absolute rarity.
b) An increased incidence is found in certain population groups, especially those of Asian descent.
c) Benign tumors and tumor-like formations are common and found in up to 50% of the population.
d) The risk of developing Kaposi's sarcoma is 20,000 times higher in HIV patients compared to normal patients.
e) Primary angiosarcoma of the aorta can be the cause of an aortic occlusion.

Answers

a) **Correct.** Vascular tumors are an extremely rare disease. They have an annual incidence of 1–2 per 10 million inhabitants and account for about 1% of malignant soft tissue tumors. Consequently, the field of vascular surgery (in contrast to visceral or bone surgery) has little to do with tumor diseases.
b) **Incorrect.** Due to the rarity of the disease, it is very difficult to identify specific risk groups. Only for certain acquired tumor entities can at-risk groups be specified. For example, in HIV-associated Kaposi's sarcoma and radiation-induced angiosarcoma after breast cancer (Stewart-Treves syndrome). According to current knowledge, there is no confirmation that certain population groups are more frequently affected.

S. Regus, *Vascular Surgery: Questions and Answers*,
https://doi.org/10.1007/978-3-662-73387-5_15

c) **Correct.** Tumor-like formations are common and found in up to 50% of the population. These are mostly hemangiomas (also known as blood sponges or strawberry marks) in the skin and superficial connective tissue, which are generally benign. Often, no further therapy is indicated; in cases of progressive enlargement, laser, cryotherapy, or surgical resection may be necessary.
d) **Correct.** Kaposi's sarcoma is a disease frequently observed in HIV patients, attributable to acquired immunodeficiency and T-cell defect. It is therefore also referred to as one of the so-called "AIDS-defining illnesses." Compared to other immunodeficiency diseases, HIV patients have an approximately 300-fold increased risk of disease.
e) **Correct.** In rare cases, a primary angiosarcoma can be the cause of an aortic occlusion. Therefore, in cases of unclear findings and atypical occlusive processes, a histological examination of the occluded vessel and the thrombotic material should always be performed. Some surgeons routinely take aortic tissue for histological assessment; however, the proportion of malignant diseases in aortic occlusion is very low and is estimated at < 1 ‰.

Question

2. Which statements about the classification of vascular tumors are correct?

a) Vascular tumors are classified as benign, locally aggressive, and malignant tumors.
b) Most benign tumors are congenital.
c) Kaposi's sarcoma originates from the endothelium.
d) Paraganglioma of the carotid body is a highly malignant and usually inoperable tumor.
e) Leiomyomas are the most common venous tumors.

Answers

a) **Correct.** Locally aggressive tumors are also referred to as borderline tumors because they grow rapidly and infiltratively but have not yet metastasized. Examples of benign tumors are hemangiomas, of borderline tumors Kaposi's sarcoma, and of malignant tumors angiosarcoma.
b) **Correct.** Hemangioma is an embryonal tumor that occurs in 1–3% of all newborns. In premature infants, it is significantly more common at 10%.
c) **Correct.** The sarcoma first described in 1872 by Moriz Kaposi, a Hungarian dermatologist, and named after him, belongs to the malignant endothelial carcinomas and is frequently localized in the skin and mucous

membranes, as well as associated with immunodeficiency (HIV) and human herpesvirus 8 (HHV 8).

d) **Incorrect.** The tumor of the carotid body is usually benign and, as a rule, has not yet metastasized. However, the metastasis rate is up to 10%, and in extensive cases with infiltration of adjacent tissue, complete resection of the carotid bifurcation may be necessary.
e) **Correct.** The veins in the pelvic and leg region are most commonly affected, almost exclusively in women. They grow slowly and become symptomatic as painless swelling once they reach a certain size. Sometimes, venous thrombosis also develops. After complete resection, recurrence is very rare, and additional therapy is therefore not necessary.

Question

3. Which statements about the diagnosis of vascular tumor diseases are correct?

a) Vascular tumor diseases are diagnosed less by the tumor itself and more by complications.
b) Ultrasound is not a suitable diagnostic tool for detecting vascular tumors.
c) Intravascular ultrasound (IVUS) can provide information about infiltration of perivascular tissue.
d) Angiography using DSA technique, unlike MRA, is of no significance today.
e) MRI can visualize both the tumor tissue and its infiltration.

Answers

a) **Correct.** Typical complications of vascular tumor diseases are:
   I. Local swelling
   II. Redness/induration
   III. Aneurysm
   IV. Peripheral embolization

   The majority of vascular tumor diseases become clinically symptomatic for the first time due to complications, not the tumor itself. Although only about 1% of embolic occlusions are caused by tumor diseases, histological examination of the embolus is generally recommended, especially in cases of atypical clinical symptoms.
b) **Incorrect.** In the hands of an experienced examiner, ultrasound is very sensitive in diagnosing vascular tumors. Especially in duplex mode, hyperperfused or hypervascularized tissue areas can be morphologically visualized. For

superficial tumors, ultrasound is a more suitable examination method than MRA; in deeper locations (abdomen, thorax), problems may arise depending on location and examination conditions. Therefore, the sensitivity of ultrasound is inferior to MR imaging in certain locations.

c) **Correct.** IVUS is suitable for visualizing tumor tissue within the vessel and its extent. 12.5 to 17.5 MHz probes are used, which are introduced percutaneously. Thus, it is an invasive diagnostic method, but without radiation exposure. Another advantage of IVUS is the possibility of taking a biopsy via the access.
d) **Incorrect.** DSA has not lost its significance as a preoperative diagnostic tool and is strictly required by most surgeons before surgical tumor resection with curative intent. Only in this way can the peripheral outflow situation be visualized and optimal reconstruction procedures planned. This is especially true for repeat procedures.
e) **Correct.** MRI is the diagnostic tool of choice for assessing the extent and characteristics of tumor tissue, as well as its infiltration. Especially in the joint area and when neural structures are involved, MRI is "unbeatable"; if necessary, the contrast agent gadolinium must be administered for more precise assessment of the vascular situation. However, for evaluating the native vessels in the outflow of the extremities, MRA is usually inferior to DSA, so for extremity involvement and before bypass reconstruction, selective angiography of the peripheral vessels should complete the preoperative diagnostics.

Question

4. Which statements about Kaposi's sarcoma are correct?

a) Kaposi's sarcoma is caused by a human herpesvirus.
b) Kaposi's sarcoma occurs only on the skin.
c) Kaposi's sarcoma is a so-called "AIDS-defining condition" and occurs only in HIV-positive patients.
d) Kaposi's sarcoma is an angioproliferative tumor.
e) The primary treatment for Kaposi's sarcoma is surgical.

Answers

a) **Correct.** The cause of Kaposi's sarcoma is human herpesvirus 8 (HHV-8). It is mainly transmitted through sexual contact, but also from an affected mother to the unborn child or during birth. Kaposi's sarcoma was first described in

1872 by Austrian dermatologist Moriz Kaposi and referred to as idiopathic pigmented sarcoma. Melanosarcoma was also a common term for a time.

b) **Incorrect.** Although Kaposi's sarcoma most often first manifests and becomes visible on the skin, mucous membranes and internal organs can also be affected. Common manifestations include the mucous membranes in the oral area, especially the gums.

c) **Incorrect.** Although Kaposi's sarcoma is still referred to as an "AIDS-defining illness," it also occurs in HIV-negative patients. Here, mainly patients with congenital or, much more commonly, acquired immunodeficiency are affected. For example, patients after organ transplantation are another risk group for Kaposi's sarcoma. In these patients, internal organs are often affected first, making diagnosis more challenging and usually taking longer.

d) **Correct.** In Kaposi's sarcoma, there is proliferation of endothelial cells, usually of skin and mucosal tissue. It is a malignant and rapidly growing tumor.

e) **Incorrect.** Treatment of Kaposi's sarcoma consists, on the one hand, of radiation therapy, and on the other, treatment of the underlying disease is essential. Thus, in HIV-positive patients, therapy of the immunodeficiency and the underlying disease is the priority. In patients with acquired immunodeficiency, for example after organ transplantation, the dosage of immunosuppression should be reviewed and, if possible, reduced. However, this should be done without endangering the organ transplant.

Question

5. Which statements about carotid body glomus tumor are correct?

a) The glomus tumor is also called a paraganglioma.
b) About 30% of carotid body tumors are malignant.
c) Since the carotid body tumor is benign, conservative management is generally recommended for small asymptomatic tumors.
d) Since paragangliomas are benign tumors, the survival rate after surgical therapy is unrestricted.
e) The carotid body tumor is highly vascularized and well visualized in imaging.

Answers

a) **Correct.** Glomus tumors are also referred to as paragangliomas. A paraganglion is a knot-like cluster of neuroendocrine cells that do not transmit their transmitters to other nerve cells, but release them directly into the bloodstream. Paraganglia are thus junctions between the autonomic nervous system and the endocrine hormonal system. Transmitters are acetylcholine (parasympathetic paraganglia = non-chromaffin) and catecholamines (sympathetic ganglia = chromaffin).

b) **Correct.** Although glomus tumors are usually benign and locally limited in growth, they metastasize in about 30% of cases. From this point, they are by definition malignant tumors with a significant risk of recurrence, even if they can be locally well resected and removed with sufficient safety margin.
c) **Incorrect.** Even though carotid paraganglioma (glomus tumor) is benign and non-infiltrative in most cases, invasive therapy is indicated early. This is due to the potential risk of metastasis in more than 30% of cases and the good surgical accessibility. In addition, for small lesions without local compression symptoms, interventional therapy (embolization) can also be successfully performed. However, it should be mentioned that most carotid body tumors are diagnosed at an advanced stage with corresponding size, so the question of interventional or even conservative therapy often does not arise.
d) **Incorrect.** In completely resected paragangliomas without metastasis, there is indeed no reduction in life expectancy compared to the general population. However, if metastasis is present at the time of diagnosis and therapy, even with tumor-free resection margins and complete removal of the malignant process, life expectancy is reduced to 5 years after diagnosis.
e) **Correct.** Paragangliomas are well and strongly vascularized and therefore always well visualized in contrast-enhanced imaging. Based on location, morphology, and pronounced vascularization, this tumor entity can be easily recognized and diagnosed. However, it should be emphasized again that this is not a vascular, but a neuroendocrine tumor. The overlap with the field of vascular surgery is not due to the origin of the tumor cells, but to the location at the carotid bulb. In most hospitals, treatment of these tumors is performed by ENT specialists. Usually, vascular surgery is only involved in large tumors requiring vascular replacement (carotid interposition graft).

Question

6. Which statements about angiosarcoma are correct?

a) Angiosarcoma is a highly malignant tumor.
b) Hemangiosarcomas of the breast show an increasing incidence.
c) Hemangiosarcomas of the liver are usually asymptomatic.

d) Angiosarcoma is one of the most common soft tissue sarcomas.
e) Hemangiosarcoma is a common malignant tumor of the heart.

Answers

a) **Correct.** Angiosarcoma is a malignant tumor that arises from the endothelial cells of blood vessels. It is a special form of soft tissue sarcoma and is classified into hemangiosarcomas (arising from the endothelial cells of blood vessels) and lymphangiosarcomas (arising from the endothelial cells of lymphatic vessels). They are most commonly found in the skin, breast, liver, and spleen. On the skin, hemangiosarcomas appear as reddish-brown spots that rapidly increase in size and may ulcerate. In the breast, angiosarcomas are often nodular and also rapidly growing.
b) **Correct.** Hemangiosarcomas in the breast area show an increasing incidence, which is related to the increase in breast-conserving therapies for breast cancer. Hemangiosarcomas of the breast occur particularly in previously operated and irradiated areas, which explains the increase in cases.
c) **Incorrect.** Since hemangiosarcoma is a highly malignant and rapidly growing tumor, it usually becomes symptomatic quickly and early. Hemangiosarcomas of the liver grow expansively and quickly reach enormous sizes. Initially, patients report B symptoms (weight loss, fatigue, night sweats), which are rather nonspecific. Specific symptoms often include upper abdominal pain and jaundice, which provide early clues to the correct diagnosis. However, a definitive diagnosis can only be made after biopsy and histological examination. The main organs affected by hemangiosarcomas are the liver and spleen.
d) **Incorrect.** Angiosarcoma is a very rare malignancy and accounts for about 1–2% of soft tissue sarcomas. Soft tissue sarcomas have an annual incidence of 2 per 100,000 inhabitants, with leiomyosarcoma being the most common. This arises from smooth muscle, e.g., the uterus.
e) **Incorrect.** Hemangiosarcoma is a rare malignant tumor arising from vascular endothelium. A typical location of this malignant soft tissue sarcoma is the heart, especially the right atrium. At least, most case reports of cardiac hemangiosarcomas involve the right heart. Therapy always includes complete tumor resection followed by chemotherapy, but the prognosis is very poor. Often, curative resection is no longer possible in advanced tumor stages, and metastasis has already occurred in most cases. Palliative chemotherapy is usually survived for only a few months.

Question

7. Which statements about paraneoplastic diseases in vascular surgery are correct?

a) Trousseau's syndrome describes paraneoplastic thrombosis in malignant tumor diseases.
b) Phlegmasia alba refers to embolism of tumor tissue in atrial myxoma.
c) Idiopathic thrombosis is the most common paraneoplastic disease in vascular surgery.
d) Raynaud's phenomenon can, in rare cases, also occur as part of a paraneoplastic syndrome.
e) A newly developed peripheral polyneuropathy can be paraneoplastic in origin.

Answers

a) **Correct.** Trousseau's syndrome, named after its first describer Armand Trousseau (1801–1867), describes thrombosis induced by malignant tumor diseases and is thus classified as a paraneoplastic syndrome. The mechanisms are not yet fully understood, but a characteristic feature is thrombosis that is not located in the immediate vicinity of the tumor or its metastases. Rather, the tumor itself or tumor-induced processes lead to the release of procoagulant signaling substances. These include, among others, tumor tissue thromboplastin, fibrinogen, and plasminogen activator inhibitor (PAI).
b) **Incorrect.** Phlegmasia alba is a synonym for Trousseau's syndrome and describes the clinical appearance of arterial embolism or thrombosis, i.e., pain and pallor. Here, too, increased blood coagulability plays the main role, not the embolization of tumor cells.
c) **Correct.** Thrombosis is the most common tumor-associated vascular disease and affects both the arterial and venous systems. Venous thromboses are much more common than arterial ones in paraneoplastic syndrome. This may be due to additional stasis in the venous system, which, together with paraneoplastic increased coagulation activity, could make the venous system more susceptible to thrombotic complications. Superficial veins are particularly affected, in the form of thrombophlebitis migrans or saltans.
d) **Correct.** Newly developed acral discoloration and pain can be interpreted as secondary Raynaud's syndrome and may be the first clinical sign of a malignant tumor disease. There are very few case reports of secondary

Raynaud's syndrome in malignant diseases, with pulmonary tumors being the most frequently mentioned. Therefore, in cases of secondary Raynaud's syndrome and corresponding risk factors (nicotine abuse and B symptoms), a chest X-ray should always be performed to diagnose or rule out pulmonary masses at an early stage.

e) **Correct.** Peripheral polyneuropathy is the most common neurological sign of a paraneoplastic syndrome. Not infrequently, patients with polyneuropathy present to vascular surgery to further clarify a vascular cause of the symptoms. If a normal vascular status with triphasic signals to the foot is found and diabetes mellitus (especially diabetic microangiopathy) is excluded, a paraneoplastic syndrome should be considered in the differential diagnosis. Since bronchial carcinoma most frequently leads to a paraneoplastic syndrome, a chest X-ray should also be performed in patients at risk with unexplained peripheral polyneuropathy.

GPSR Compliance

The European Union's (EU) General Product Safety Regulation (GPSR) is a set of rules that requires consumer products to be safe and our obligations to ensure this.

If you have any concerns about our products, you can contact us on ProductSafety@springernature.com

In case Publisher is established outside the EU, the EU authorized representative is:

Springer Nature Customer Service Center GmbH
Europaplatz 3
69115 Heidelberg, Germany

Batch number: 10723247

Printed by Printforce, the Netherlands